Color
Atlas of
Dermatology

Color Atlas of Dermatology

JEFFREY P. CALLEN, MD
Professor of Medicine (Dermatology)
Chief, Division of Dermatology
University of Louisville School of Medicine
Louisville, KY

KENNETH E. GREER, MD
Chairman, Dermatology Department
University of Virginia Health Sciences Center
Charlottesville, VA

ANTOINETTE F. HOOD, MD
Professor
Departments of Dermatology and Pathology
Indiana University
Indianapolis, IN

AMY S. PALLER, MD
Departments of Pediatrics and Dermatology
The Children's Memorial Hospital
Northwestern University Medical School
Chicago, IL

LEONARD J. SWINYER, MD
Clinical Professor of Dermatology
Division of Dermatology
University of Utah
Salt Lake City, UT

W.B. SAUNDERS COMPANY
A Division of Harcourt Brace & Company
Philadelphia   London   Toronto   Montreal   Sydney   Tokyo

W.B. SAUNDERS COMPANY
A Division of
Harcourt Brace & Company

The Curtis Center
Independence Square West
Philadelphia, Pennsylvania 19106

Library of Congress Cataloging-in-Publication Data

Color atlas of dermatology / Jeffrey P. Callen . . . [et al.].

p.   cm.

Includes index.

ISBN 0–7216–3756–6

1. Dermatology—Atlases.   I. Callen, Jeffrey P.
    [DNLM: 1. Skin Diseases—atlases.   WR 17 C7183 1993]

RL81.C655 1993

616.5′0022′2—dc20

DNLM/DLC   93–10914

Color Atlas of Dermatology   ISBN 0–7216–3756–6

Printed in the United States of America.

Last digit is the print number: 9   8   7   6   5   4   3   2   1

FOREWORD

How dull, uninteresting, and devoid of challenge it would be if dermatologic diagnosis were as simple as the identification of birds. My field guide states that the belted kingfisher "is our only blue bird that dives in the water," that the bank swallow is "our only swallow with a white throat and brown breastband." Not so easy with dermatitis herpetiformis and pilomatricoma. Numerous atlases and textbooks of dermatology have approached the challenge of how to name and characterize the diseases we deal with daily.

Atlases take the position that images and their organization can convey information in a manner complementary to and perhaps better than mere words. The term "atlas" in reference to a book was first applied to Mercator's collection of maps in 1636, which contains a picture of the Titan Atlas supporting the heavens. In the nineteenth century, the term atlas was applied to similar books with extensive illustrative plates on a variety of topics.

Dermatologic atlases have been extremely popular usually because of the quality of their graphics. Among the most famous is that of Duhring, *Atlas of Skin Disease* (1876–1880). The original engravings from the Duhring *Atlas* decorate the walls of the Department of Dermatology at the University of Pennsylvania. It is a delight to watch visiting dermatologists carefully examine the picture and pit their diagnostic acumen against the diagnosis of 120 years ago.

Atlases are a snapshot of reality. They are not the distillate of experience and other written works. They contain the original data, from real patients. As such, they are valuable for the present and also for the future. As we learn about the molecular mechanisms of health and disease, we can look back at the raw clinical data with new eyes. There is special exhilaration looking at an old atlas to view those patients and their diseases with a new paradigm. This is part of the truth and power in the Chinese proverb, "one picture is worth more than ten thousand words."

This atlas is produced by an energetic, imaginative, and committed group of dermatologists who have taken their mission as medical educators seriously. They have assembled an outstanding collection of photographs, which is the essence of any atlas. The efforts in the assembling of these photographs we understand well, as we went through a similar process in our *Diagnosis of Skin Disease*. The authors have measured up to the high standards they set for themselves. They have included a vade mecum of useful charts and tables.

In addition to being a valuable atlas for the present, it is one that should be put in the time capsule so our dermatologic great-grandchildren can see what we called the diseases of our time.

LOWELL A. GOLDSMITH, MD, ROCHESTER, NY
GERALD S. LAZARUS, MD, PHILADELPHIA, PA

PREFACE

Our impetus for producing the *Atlas of Dermatology* has been based on our collective desire to teach. In this work we have divided cutaneous disorders by morphology, configuration, or distribution. This simulates the nature in which patients are seen in our offices, hospitals, or clinics. The patient generally presents to us with the desire for diagnosis and treatment. It is the former that this work addresses.

The book is divided into sections that are not necessarily of equal length. We have minimized the text in order to maximize the number and variety of photographs that could be presented. The text consists of either tables of differential diagnoses or legends for the figures. Thus, if readers can describe a skin lesion, they can review a group of photographs of diseases that could be responsible for the observed lesions. There is no particular order to the lesions presented in any section. We have not alphabetized the diseases, as many have several names, and we have not attempted to place them in order of frequency, since no universal agreement exists.

The reader may note that there is overlap among morphologic categories. This approaches reality, since many diseases can have a multitude of expressions. Also, as diseases evolve, their manifestations may change, and thus at any one moment in this evolutionary process a different manifestation is possible. Lesions change from blisters to erosions, from vesicles to pustules, and from papules to nodules to tumors, to name only a few examples. Thus, it is necessary in some instances to allow time to aid in final diagnosis. Furthermore, the reader may note that some entities or variants are not represented. These representative photographs were carefully chosen to most closely parallel all common and some rare skin disorders seen in North America.

We hope the use of this book will make readers better able to diagnose their patients' cutaneous disease.

ACKNOWLEDGMENTS

Many of our colleagues have aided us in obtaining the excellent photographs contained in this Atlas. Through the last 15 years, the principal authors have traded slides with a variety of dermatologists across the United States and Canada. We have clearly indicated which photographs are not those of the authors. We apologize to any of our colleagues whom we may not have correctly acknowledged. Also, we would like to thank our families, who have been supportive of our efforts. Lastly, we thank Ms. Sandra Lingle, who has coordinated the production of this text from our offices in Louisville.

We specifically acknowledge the contributions of Dr. Chris Baker[1] of Melbourne, Australia; Dr. Fernando Botero[2] of Naples, Florida; Dr. Joseph Chanda[3] of Melbourne, Florida; Dr. Steve Estes[4] of Cincinnati, Ohio; Dr. Neil Fenske[5] of Tampa, Florida; Dr. Loren Golitz[6] of Denver, Colorado; Dr. Ruth Hanno[7] of Tampa, Florida; Dr. Donald Hazelrigg[6] of Evansville, Indiana; Dr. Paul Lucky[9] of Cincinnati, Ohio; Dr. William Parsley[10] of Louisville, Kentucky; Dr. Neil Penneys[11] of Saint Louis, Missouri; Dr. Robert Soderstrom[12] of Flint, Michigan; Dr. Mary Spraker[13] of Atlanta, Georgia; Dr. Marek Stawiski[14] of Grand Rapids, Michigan; Dr. Richard Sturm[15] of Atlanta, Georgia; Dr. Mark Unis[16] of Fort Lauderdale, Florida; and Dr. John Zone[17] of Salt Lake City, Utah. The superscript numbers by their names have been used throughout this volume to identify the slides they have been kind enough to allow us to use.

CONTENTS

INTRODUCTION

DEFINITIONS AND INTRODUCTION

In the specialty of dermatology, the physical examination of the skin, its appendages, and the mucous membranes forms the cornerstone of diagnosis. Proper examination often leads the examiner to obtain appropriate historical information or to select appropriate laboratory tests that are confirmatory.

In order to examine the skin properly, patients must expose an adequate amount of surface. Proper illumination of surface is essential, and physicians must be prepared to observe the changes in front of them.

Natural lighting, although ideal for cutaneous examination, is often impossible to obtain in an office or hospital room. Bright overhead fluorescent lighting is preferred to incandescent or indirect lighting. Additional tools which may be useful for the examination include a simple, but bright, penlight or small flashlight for side lighting of a lesion. Also, a variety of magnifying lenses with fluorescent rings may be attached to the examination room wall or wheeled independently. A new instrument is the epiluminescence scope, which may prove valuable in predicting whether a pigmented lesion is benign or malignant. The instrument is small and can easily be carried to the hospital room. The physical examination is largely dependent on inspection, but the skin lesion should also be palpated. Most skin lesions are not contagious, but in today's environment with the high prevalence of skin disease associated with human immunodeficiency virus (HIV), it is prudent to consider using gloves for most examinations and all procedures. The purpose of palpation of the lesion is to assess its texture and consistency. Palpation can also determine whether the lesion blanches, whether there is edema in the area, and whether the lesion is tender.

The examination then consists of several components that are addressed in this Atlas separately. Cornerstones of dermatologic diagnosis are (1) the morphology of the lesion, (2) the configuration of the lesion, and (3) the distribution of the lesion. The foremost task is determining the morphology of the lesion(s), since this will begin the process of differential diagnosis. In this first section of our Atlas, we will define the terms used for description of morphology, configuration, and distribution. Each subsequent section will deal with individual morphologic terms. Thus, as an examiner of the skin, if you can learn to observe and correctly assess these three characteristics, you will be able to review classic examples of the diseases within the appropriate section.

DEFINITIONS

The components of the skin are as follows:

The *epidermis* is the outer layer of the skin and is divided into four layers: the basal cell layer, the stratum spinosum, the stratum granulosum, and the stratum corneum. The epidermis also contains melanocytes and Langerhans cells. The latter serve as an important part of the skin's immune system.

The *dermis* is the support structure for the epidermis. This layer contains blood vessels, nerves, and appendages. It is composed of collagen, elastic fibers, and ground substance. The dermis is divided into two layers: the papillary dermis (uppermost portion) and the reticular dermis.

Skin appendages are the eccrine sweat glands, the sebaceous glands, the hair, and the nails.

Subcutaneous fat layer. Nerves and blood vessels course through this layer.

Dermal-epidermal junction. This complex area is the interface between these two layers.

MORPHOLOGIC LESIONS

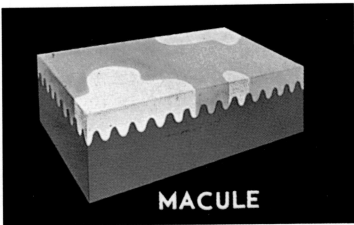

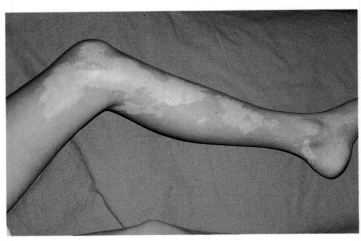

1.1
A, Schematic diagram of a *macule,* which is a flat, nonpalpable skin lesion, recognizable only by virtue of a different color from the surrounding skin. Macules come in white (hypopigmented), brown, blue, black, or yellow (pigmented) or red or purple (erythematous or purpuric) varieties. (From Caplan RM, Kopf AW, Sulzberger MB: Skin Lesions Depicted and Defined. By permission from the Sulzberger Institute for Dermatologic Communication and Education and the American Academy of Dermatology.) *B,* Vitiligo. Sharply demarcated white *macules.*

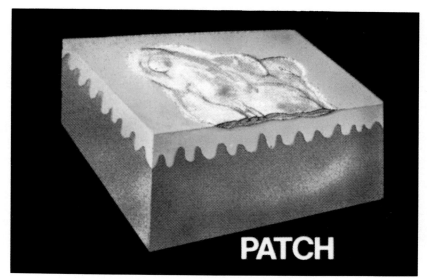

A

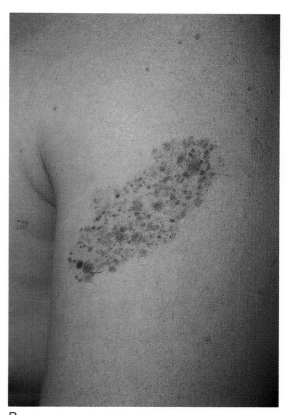

B

1.2

A, Schematic diagram of a *patch.* A large macule that may have some subtle surface change, such as fine scale or fine wrinkling. While the consistency of the surface is altered, the lesion itself is not palpable. (From Lookingbill DP, Marks JG Jr: Principles of Dermatology. WB Saunders Co, Philadelphia, 1986, p. 29.) *B,* Nevus spilus. This speckled, pigmented area is a large macule or patch. In this case there was no demonstrable surface change.

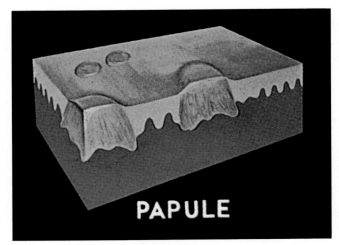

A

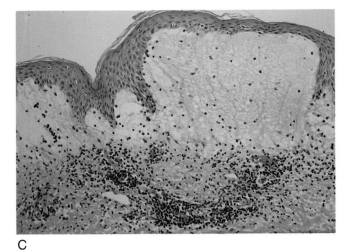

B

1.3

A, Schematic diagram of a *papule,* a small, elevated skin lesion usually under 0.5 cm in diameter. Papules are about equal in diameter and depth. They may have accompanying surface changes such as scale. (From Caplan RM, Kopf AW, Sulzberger MB: Skin Lesions Depicted and Defined. By permission from the Sulzberger Institute for Dermatologic Communication and Education and the American Academy of Dermatology.) *B,* Polymorphous light eruption. Multiple erythematous papules on the sun-exposed surface of the arm. *C,* The histologic change shown correlates well with the schematic and clinical photographs. Marked dermal edema with a perivascular lymphocytic infiltrate is present. Dilated vessels account for some of the erythema.

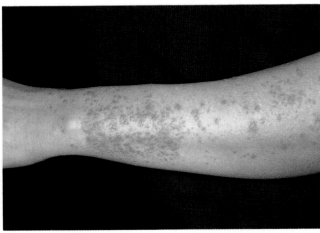

C

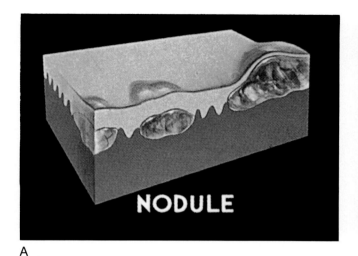

A

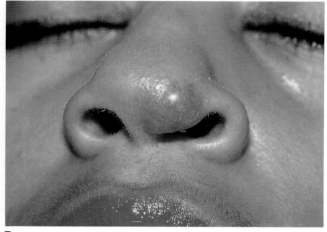

B

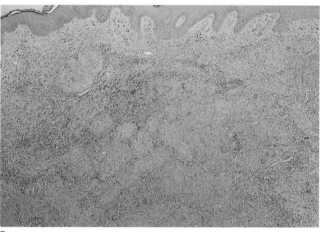

C

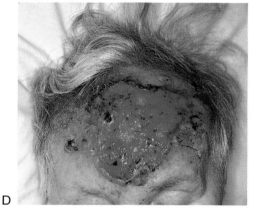

D

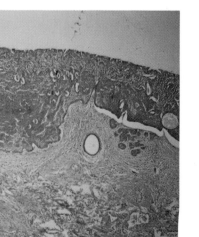

E

1.4

A, Schematic diagram of a *nodule,* an elevated lesion greater than 0.5 cm in both width and depth. Papules, if they are neoplastic, will grow to become nodules, and if left in place, lesions that are nodules can grow to become *tumors.* The size differences are arbitrary. Nodules and tumors may represent inflammatory diseases or may be representative of neoplastic processes. (From Caplan RM, Kopf AW, Sulzberger MB: Skin Lesions Depicted and Defined. By permission from the Sulzberger Institute for Dermatologic Communication and Education and the American Academy of Dermatology.) *B,* Sarcoidosis. This patient has an erythematous *nodule* along the nasal rim. There is no surface change, but there are telangiectasias within the lesion. *C,* Histopathology of sarcoidosis reveals a noncaseating granuloma with multinucleated giant cells in the dermis. The epidermis is normal. *D,* A large basal cell carcinoma is representative of a *tumor.* This tumor grew slowly over more than 10 years from a papule to a nodule to an ulcerating tumor. *E,* Histopathology of a small basal cell carcinoma. Note the normal epidermis laterally, with an ulcerated surface over the tumor.

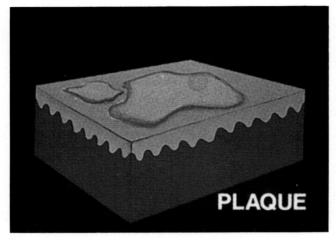

A

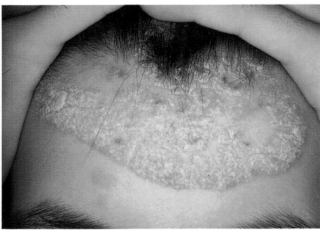

B

1.5

A, Schematic diagram of a *plaque,* an elevated, plateau-like lesion greater in its diameter than in its depth. The surface may or may not have secondary changes such as scale or crusting. Plaques can be a manifestation of an inflammatory process or a neoplastic process. They may be due to primary disease in the epidermis or dermis. (From Caplan RM, Kopf AW, Sulzberger MB: Skin Lesions Depicted and Defined. By permission from the Sulzberger Institute for Dermatologic Communication and Education and the American Academy of Dermatology.) *B,* This patient with psoriasis vulgaris demonstrates a characteristic scaly plaque. *C,* Histopathologic changes of psoriasis demonstrate the thickened epidermis with excess stratum corneum that correlates well with the clinical changes seen in *B.*

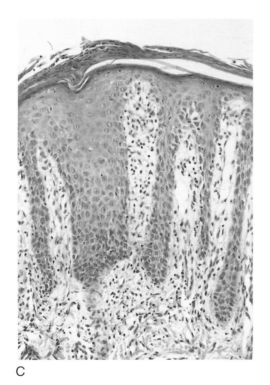

C

1.6

A, Schematic diagram of lesions that contain clear fluid. *Vesicles* are small lesions (0.5 cm in diameter), whereas *bullae* are larger lesions. These lesions represent fluid accumulation within the epidermis or at the dermal-epidermal junction. (From Caplan RM, Kopf AW, Sulzberger MB: Skin Lesions Depicted and Defined. By permission from the Sulzberger Institute for Dermatologic Communication and Education and the American Academy of Dermatology.) *B,* This patient with herpes gestationis (a pregnancy-related immunobullous disease) demonstrates both vesicles and bullae. The lesions are grouped (herpetiform: see below). One area shows a resolving blister and this represents a crusted erosion (see below). Vesicles and bullae are dynamic lesions; they become pustules and/or erosions with time. *C,* Skin biopsy from a patient with bullous pemphigoid is demonstrative of a subepidermal bulla with accumulation of fluid and inflammatory cells immediately below the epidermis.

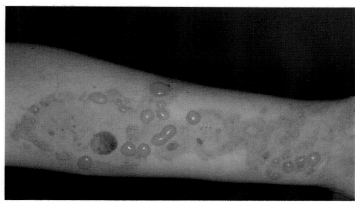

A

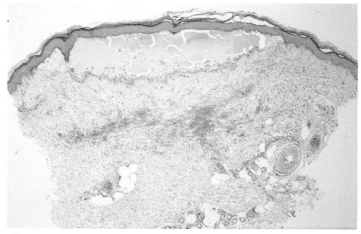

B

C

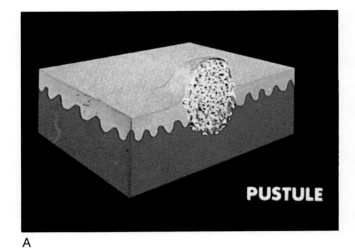

A

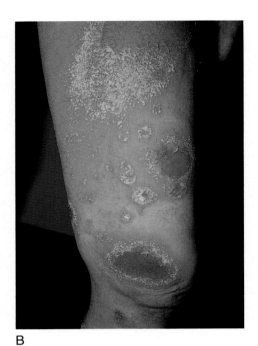

B

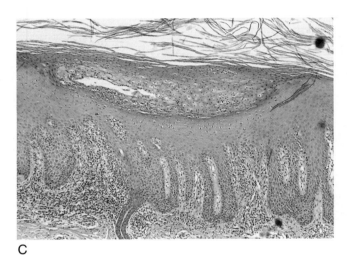

C

1.7
A, Schematic diagram of a *pustule*, a fluid-filled sack that contains cloudy or purulent material. (From Caplan RM, Kopf AW, Sulzberger MB: Skin Lesions Depicted and Defined. By permission from the Sulzberger Institute for Dermatologic Communication and Education and the American Academy of Dermatology.) *B*, Pustular psoriasis is a rare and potentially life-threatening manifestation of psoriasis characterized by sheets of small *pustules* on an erythematous base. *C*, Histopathologic examination of pustular psoriasis shows some of the changes of typical psoriasis (see Fig. 1.5C) with a massive accumulation of polymorphonuclear leukocytes in the subcorneal area of the epidermis.

1.8
A, This schematic diagram demonstrates three changes. An *erosion* is a loss of surface epidermis that is superficial and often occurs after the natural breakage of a vesicle, bulla, or papule. An *ulcer* is a loss of epidermis that extends into the dermis or subcutaneous areas and is usually as broad as it is deep. A *fissure* is a crack in the skin that is usually narrow but deep. Fissures and ulcers are often painful; erosions are merely uncomfortable. (From Caplan RM, Kopf AW, Sulzberger MB: Skin Lesions Depicted and Defined. By permission from the Sulzberger Institute for Dermatologic Communication and Education and the American Academy of Dermatology.) *B*, This patient has Hailey-Hailey disease (benign familial pemphigus), a rare inherited form of blistering disease. This disorder is most commonly manifested by erosions in the folds of the body (the axilla in this patient). Crusting is also seen. *C*, Pyoderma gangrenosum is a rare ulcerative disorder that is often a manifestation of a systemic disease. The epidermis is totally lost and, in this case, the margin is violaceous and undermined. *D*, Histopathologic examination of pyoderma gangrenosum reveals the loss of epidermis and dermal inflammation. *E*, This patient with hand eczema has cracks in the skin that represent fissures.

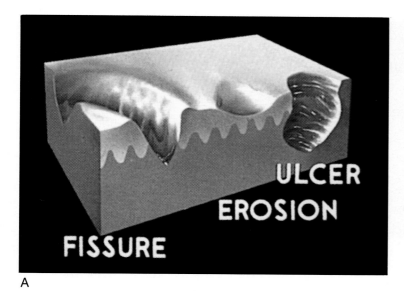

A

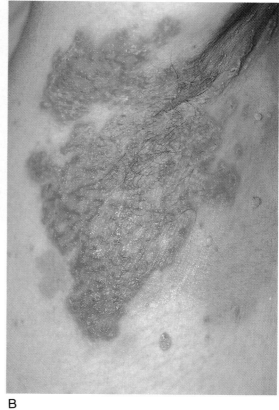

B

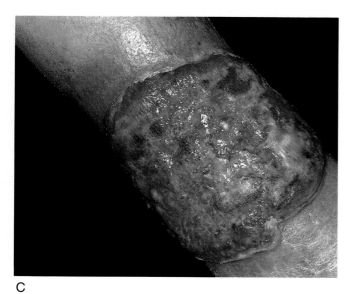

C

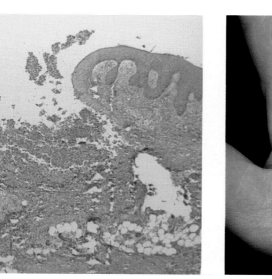

D

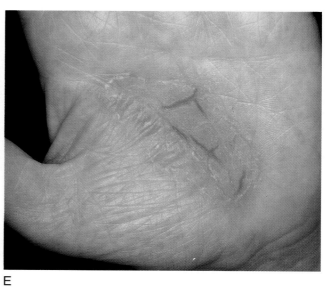

E

1.8

See legend on opposite page

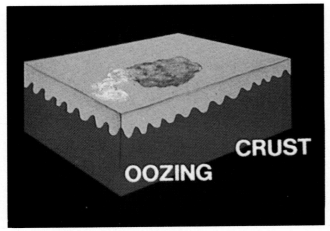

A

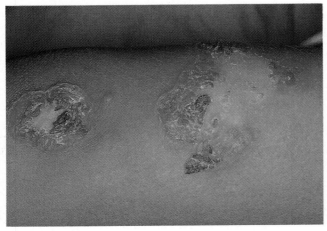

B

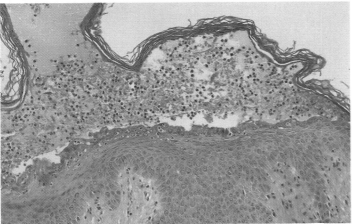

C

1.9

A, Schematic diagram of *crusting,* which occurs when serum and/or purulent material becomes dried on the surface. This is most often the result of breakage of pustules, bullae, or vesicles. (From Caplan RM, Kopf AW, Sulzberger MB: Skin Lesions Depicted and Defined. By permission from the Sulzberger Institute for Dermatologic Communication and Education and the American Academy of Dermatology.) *B,* Impetigo—erosion with golden crust. *C,* Histopathology of bullous impetigo reveals the subcorneal accumulation of purulent material. There was subcorneal leukocyte accumulation in pustular psoriasis (see Fig. 1.7*C*), but there were also other changes in the epidermis that help to distinguish these two entities.

1.10

A, Schematic diagram of a *wheal* (hive). This represents a variation on the papules or plaque in which the cause of the lesion is dermal edema. These lesions have no epidermal change, are often transient, and may have a central pallor. (From Caplan RM, Kopf AW, Sulzberger MB: Skin Lesions Depicted and Defined. By permission from the Sulzberger Institute for Dermatologic Communication and Education and the American Academy of Dermatology.) *B,* In this patient with urticaria, we were able to demonstrate the phenomenon of dermatographism, which occurs when wheals (hives) are induced after pressure. This example took place at the University of Michigan in a consenting patient on a Friday before a home football game.

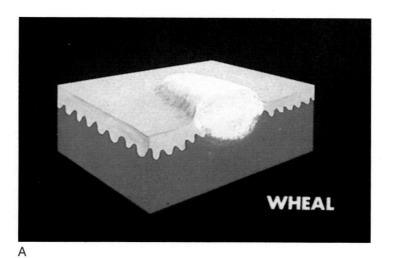

A

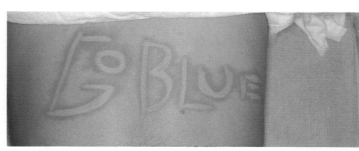

B

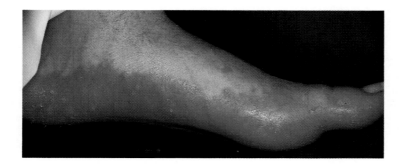

1.11

This patient with graft-versus-host disease demonstrates *erythema* of the skin. This change results from a dilation of the blood vessels in the dermis. Erythema is blanchable.[15]

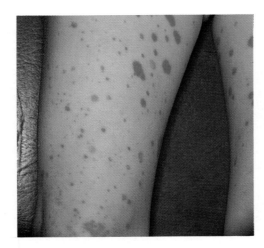

1.12
A patient with Henoch-Schönlein *purpura* demonstrates blood vessel disruption and extravasation of blood into the dermis. This lesion is nonblanchable. This particular patient has palpable (papular) purpura as opposed to a macular (nonpalpable) variant.

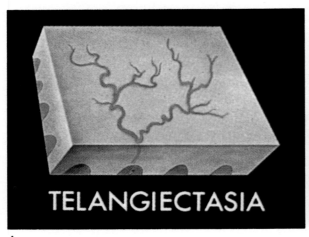

A

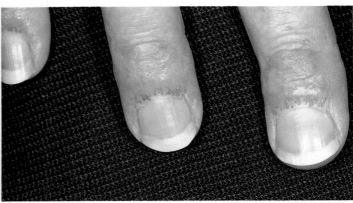

B

1.13
A, Schematic diagram of *telangiectasia.* In this case there is enlargement of the superficial blood vessel to the point of its being visible. This change also may result in blanching. (From Caplan RM, Kopf AW, Sulzberger MB: Skin Lesions Depicted and Defined. By permission from the Sulzberger Institute for Dermatologic Communication and Education and the American Academy of Dermatology.) *B,* Periungual telangiectasias in a patient with dermatomyositis.

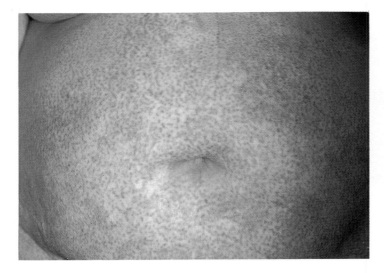

1.14
Poikiloderma is a reticulated pattern of hyperpigmentation, hypopigmentation, and erythema with telangiectasias. This patient has an entity known as poikiloderma atrophicans vasculare, which may precede the development of mycosis fungoides (a cutaneous T-cell lymphoma), may occur in collagen vascular diseases, or may be idiopathic.

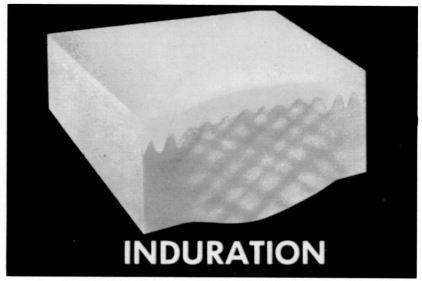

A

1.15

A, Schematic diagram of an *induration.* This change represents a dermal thickening produced by excessive dermal collagen, or by dermal infiltrative processes. The feel of the skin is often more important than visual change. (From Lookingbill DP, Marks JG Jr: Principles of Dermatology. WB Saunders Co, Philadelphia, 1986, p. 30.) *B,* Linear morphea. This child has a linear area of hardened skin that represents a localized variety of scleroderma. *C,* Histopathologic examination of linear morphea reveals a greatly thickened dermis.

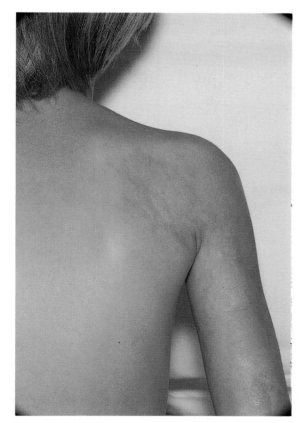

B

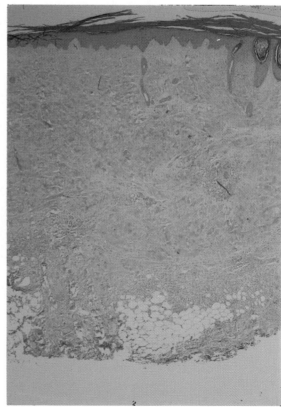

C

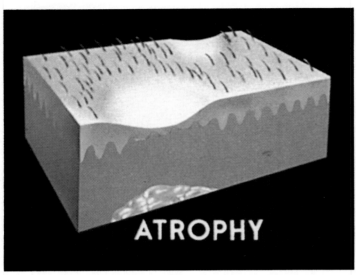

A

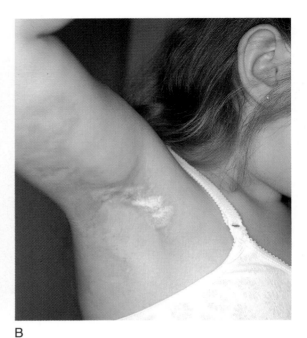

B

1.16

A, Schematic diagram depicting *atrophy,* a loss of tissue. Atrophy can be epidermal, dermal, or subcutaneous. With epidermal atrophy the skin appears thin, translucent, and/or wrinkled. With dermal or subcutaneous atrophy there is depression of the skin. (From Caplan RM, Kopf AW, Sulzberger MB: Skin Lesions Depicted and Defined. By permission from the Sulzberger Institute for Dermatologic Communication and Education and the American Academy of Dermatology.) *B,* Lichen sclerosus et atrophicus is an idiopathic condition in which epidermal atrophy is present. Note the hypopigmented, wrinkled areas.

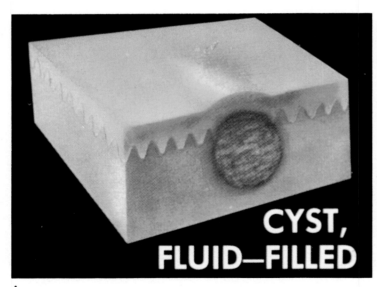

A

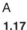

1.17

A, Schematic diagram of a *cyst,* a nodule or tumor filled with either liquid or semisolid material. A true cyst has an epithelial lining, whereas a pseudocyst is not lined. (From Lookingbill DP, Marks JG Jr: Principles of Dermatology. WB Saunders Co, Philadelphia, 1986, p. 29.) *B,* Multiple scrotal epidermal cysts are present in this patient.

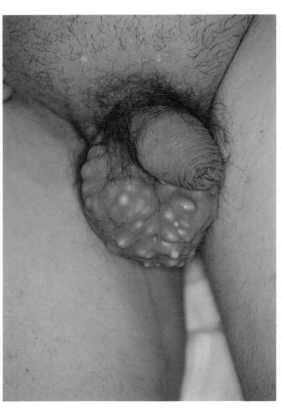

B

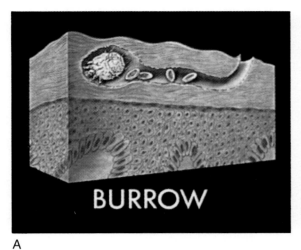

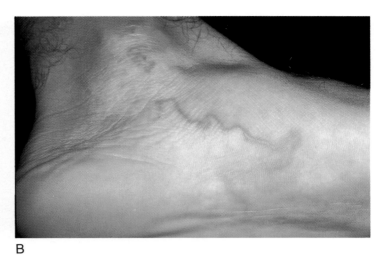

A

B

1.18

A, Schematic diagram of a *burrow.* This term refers to a tunnel caused by a burrowing organism. (From Caplan RM, Kopf AW, Sulzberger MB: Skin Lesions Depicted and Defined. By permission from the Sulzberger Institute for Dermatologic Communication and Education and the American Academy of Dermatology.) *B,* Cutaneous larva migrans. In this patient the organism gradually crawls under the surface, producing a winding *(serpiginous)* path.

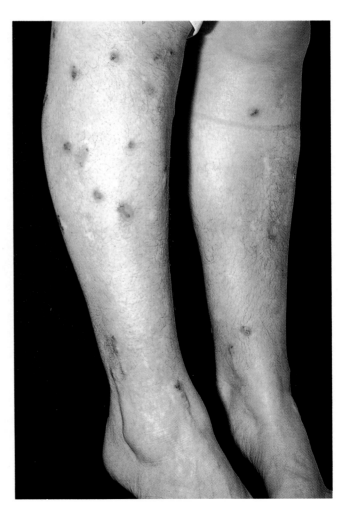

1.19

Excoriations are erosions of the skin due to external manipulation, usually by the patient's own fingernails. These lesions are frequently linear.

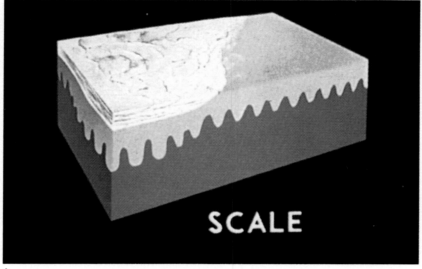

A

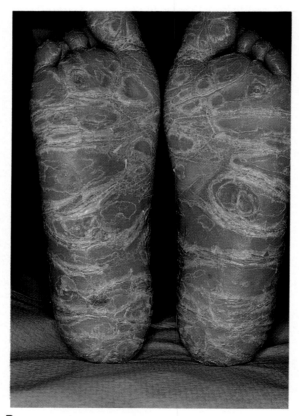

B

1.20
A, Schematic diagram representing *scale.* Scales consist of thickened stratum corneum. (From Caplan RM, Kopf AW, Sulzberger MB: Skin Lesions Depicted and Defined. By permission from the Sulzberger Institute for Dermatologic Communication and Education and the American Academy of Dermatology.) *B,* This patient has an unusual ichthyotic syndrome. Unusual scales in a geometric pattern are seen.

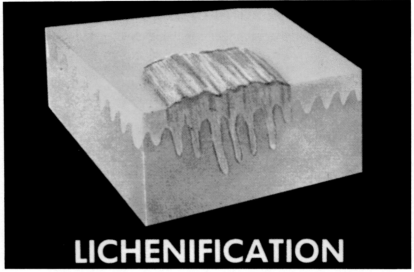

A

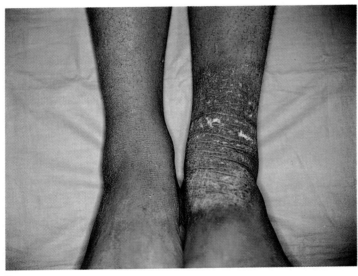

B

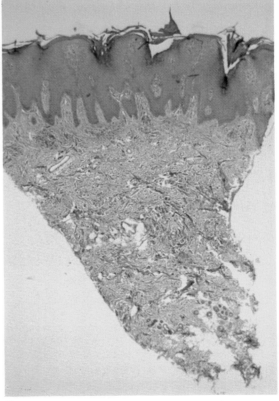

C

1.21

A, Lichenification refers to thickening of the epidermis. The skin feels thick, and its normal markings, which are usually barely visible, are greatly accentuated. (From Lookingbill DP, Marks JG Jr: Principles of Dermatology. WB Saunders Co, Philadelphia, 1986, p. 30.) *B,* Lichen simplex chronicus, which in this patient developed from chronic rubbing of the leg. The leg on the right shows marked accentuation of the skin markings.[2] *C,* Histopathologically, lichen simplex chronicus is represented by a marked epidermal thickening. Even the accentuated skin markings can be seen in this specimen.

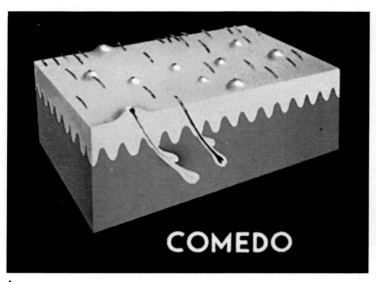

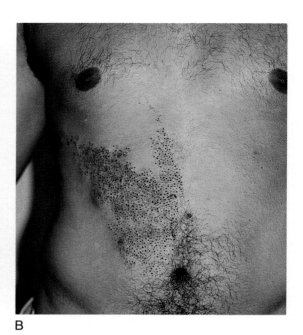

A

B

1.22

A, A *comedo* is a noninflammatory lesion in which there is keratin impaction. The most common form of comedo occurs in acne. (From Caplan RM, Kopf AW, Sulzberger MB: Skin Lesions Depicted and Defined. By permission from the Sulzberger Institute for Dermatologic Communication and Education and the American Academy of Dermatology.) *B,* Nevus comedonicus. This patient has nevoid alteration in which multiple comedones are present.

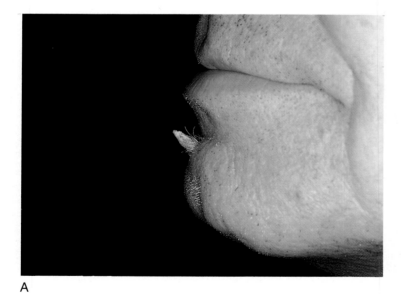

A

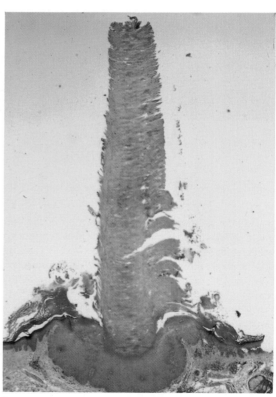

1.23

A, A cutaneous *horn*. This change is due to excessive accumulation of stratum corneum in a highly localized area. *B,* Histopathologic appearance of a cutaneous horn.

B

CONFIGURATIONS

Round Lesions

There are a variety of terms for round lesions that are used only with specific dermatologic processes. These terms include nummular and discoid. In addition, targetoid and annular lesions are often round.

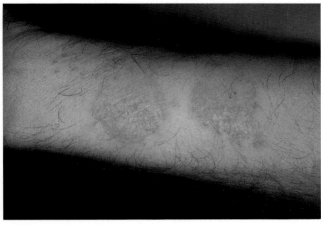

1.24
Nummular eczema. The term nummular refers to round lesions. *Eczema* comes from the Greek, meaning to boil. Eczema can be acute, represented by vesicles and bullae, or chronic, represented by lichenification.

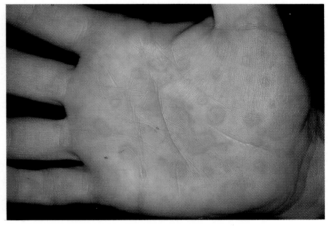

1.26
Targetoid. Round lesions in which concentric rings with color variations are present. This is relatively specific for erythema multiforme.

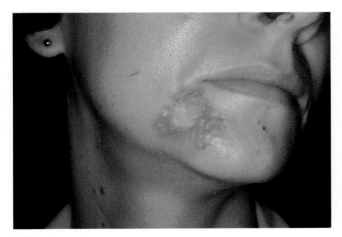

1.25
Discoid lupus erythematosus. Round or oval cutaneous lesions occurring in patients with lupus erythematosus.

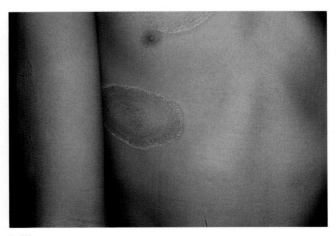

1.27
Annular. This refers to a ring-shaped lesion with an active border. The annularity may be manifested as scales along the border, or an infiltrative dermal process with an active elevated border and a clear center. This patient has erythema annulare centrifugum.

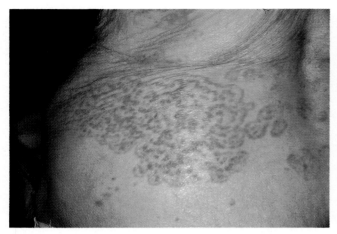

1.28

Serpiginous or *gyrate* refers to a snakelike pattern. The term *polycyclic* is also sometimes used synonomously. This patient has a condition known as erythema gyratum repens, which was a manifestation of her breast cancer.

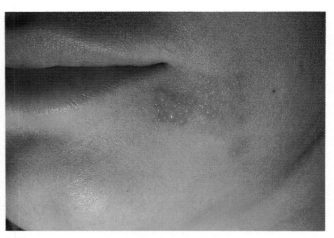

1.30

Herpetiform refers to lesions grouped in a manner similar to that seen with herpes simplex, the condition illustrated. However, this term does *not* refer to the presence of a viral infection.

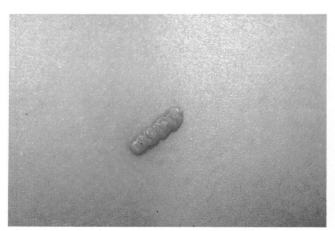

1.29

Linear is used to describe lesions that occur in a line. In this case there are multiple molluscum contagiosum lesions that have been inoculated into a traumatized area. Another term used is *koebnerized*, for *Koebner's phenomenon* in which disease develops in traumatized areas. Psoriasis and lichen planus are diseases in which Koebner's phenomenon is common.

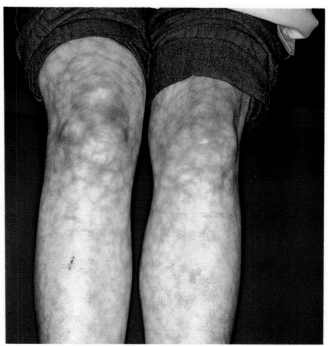

1.31

Reticular or *reticulated* describes a netlike pattern. This patient has livedo reticularis as a manifestation of lupus erythematosus.

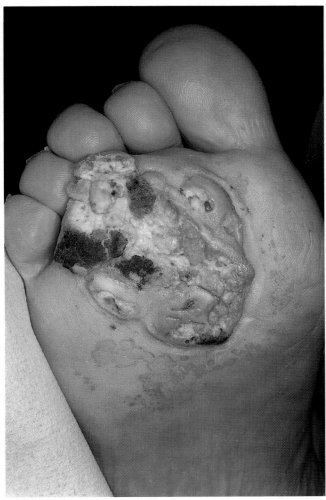

1.32
Verrucous is used to refer to a wartlike process. This patient has verrucous squamous cell carcinoma.

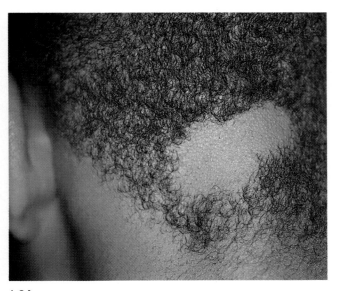

1.34
Alopecia is loss of hair. This patient has an immunologically mediated loss of hair known as alopecia areata.

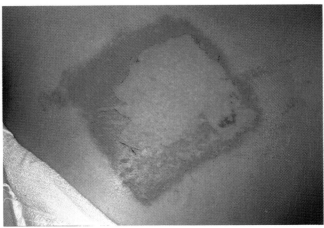

1.33
A configuration in which there are right angles suggests an external cause. In this patient the erosion with square corners is due to the application of lye, *factitiously*.

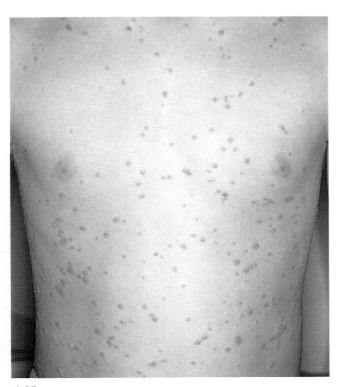

1.35
Guttate. This term means droplike and is generally used as a form of psoriasis.

DISTRIBUTIONS

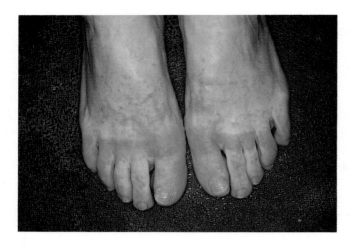

1.36

Externally induced. Contact dermatitis caused by the leather band of a sandal. Unusual configurations such as linear or square suggest an external factor.

1.37

Photodistribution. Disease induced or exacerbated by exposure to light. The disease spares protected areas.

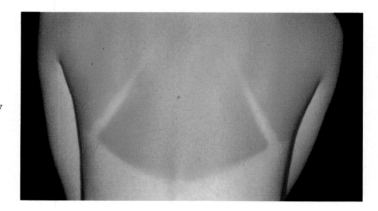

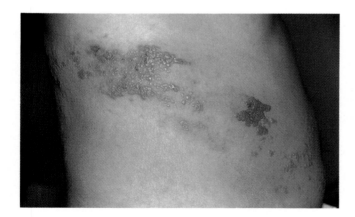

1.38

Zosteriform or *dermatomal.* Occurring within the distribution of a nerve.

Other terms used to describe a dermatologic distribution are as follows: *generalized, symmetric, flexural* or *extensor, palmoplantar, periorificial,* and *periungual.*

The following is a modification of an algorithm for diagnosis of skin disease developed by Lookingbill and Marks (Principles of Dermatology, WB Saunders Co, Philadelphia, 1986). After assessing the presence or absence of a skin problem, the following questions can be addressed. This can be used to guide the reader to an appropriate section of this Atlas.

(1) Is the lesion a growth, an eruption, and/or a pigmentary change?
  Growths:
  A. Epidermal (see papules or nodules)
  B. Dermal (see nodules)
  C. Pigmented (see macules [Chapter 2], papules, or nodules)
  Eruptions:
  A. With epidermal involvement
    1. Eczematous (see vesiculobullous or papules)
    2. Scaling (see papules)
    3. Vesiculobullous (see vesicles and bullae [Chapter 5])
    4. Papular (see papules)
    5. Pustular (see pustules or vesicles and bullae)
    6. Pigmentary changes (see macules or papules)
  B. Without epidermal involvement
    1. Red
      a. Blanchable (erythema) (see erythema or telangiectasia)
      b. Nonblanchable (purpura) (see purpura)
    2. Induration (see sclerosis)
(2) Is the lesion a pigmentary change: macular vs. palpable (see macules or papules)?
(3) Is the change seen otherwise unclassified among the previous categories (miscellaneous)?
  A. Ulcers (see Chapter 10)
  B. Atrophy (see Chapter 12)
(4) Is there a specific area of the body that is affected or is there a specific distribution?
  A. Regional disorders
    1. Hair (see Chapter 23)
    2. Nails
    3. Mucous membranes
    4. Palmoplantar
B. Distributions
    1. Photodistribution
    2. Intertriginous
    3. Generalized

CUTANEOUS PRIMARY LESIONS AND SECONDARY CHANGES

2

MACULES

Macules are flat lesions that are noticed because their color varies from the surrounding area. Patches are large macules and may have some subtle surface change. Macular lesions may be divided by color into brown or tan, white or hypopigmented, blue or red. The lesions can be further divided in relation to the predominant area affected.

BROWN MACULES

Primarily on Sun-Exposed Surfaces

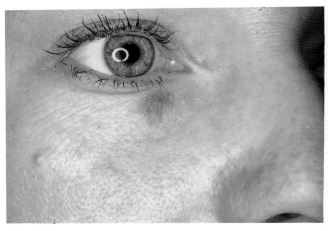

2.1
Actinic lentigo. This young woman has a tan macule under her eye.

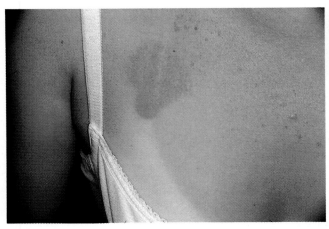

2.2
Berloque dermatitis. This hyperpigmented, irregularly shaped macule occurred as a phototoxic reaction to a psoralen-containing perfume. A similar dermatitis can occur after contact with other phototoxic chemicals.

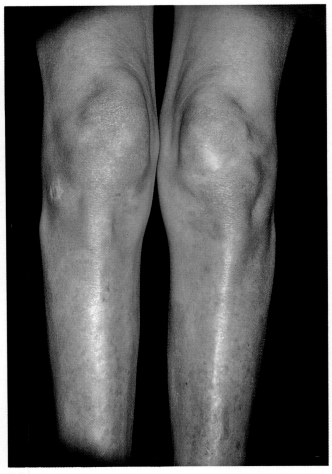

2.3
Drug-induced pigmentation. This patient developed this hyperpigmentation after ingestion of quinacrine hydrochloride.

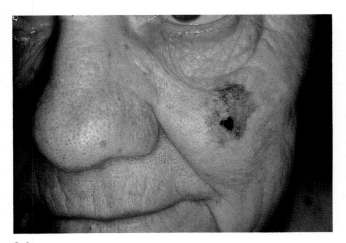

2.4
Lentigo maligna. A premalignant melanocytic neoplasm. Note the variation in pigment.

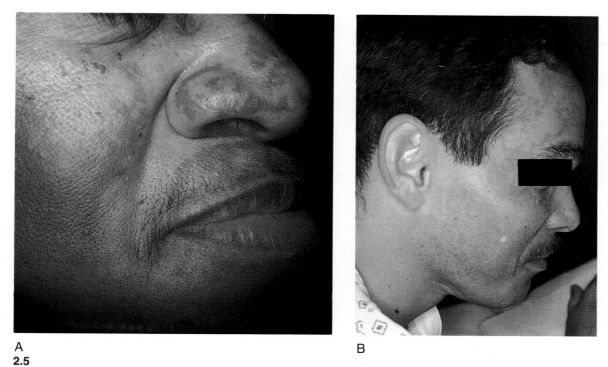

A
2.5
A, Melasma. This tan pigmentation is also known as the mask of pregnancy. *B*, Melasma is less common in males but can occasionally occur.

2.6
Xeroderma pigmentosum. Patients with this genetic disorder are unable to repair ultraviolet-damaged DNA. They freckle at an early age and eventually develop multiple cutaneous malignancies.

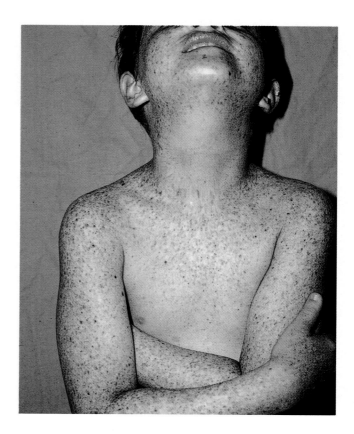

Brown Macules or Patches Not Confined to Sun-Exposed Surfaces

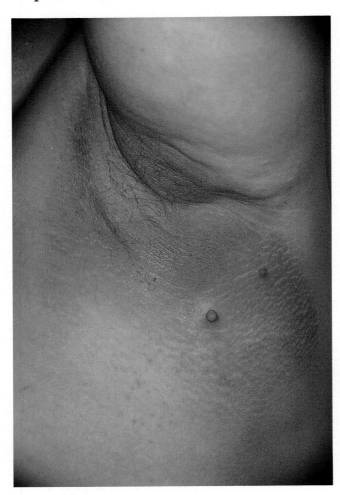

2.7
Acanthosis nigricans. Velvety patches of hyperpigmentation within the skin folds. This patient also has an infarcted skin tag.[2]

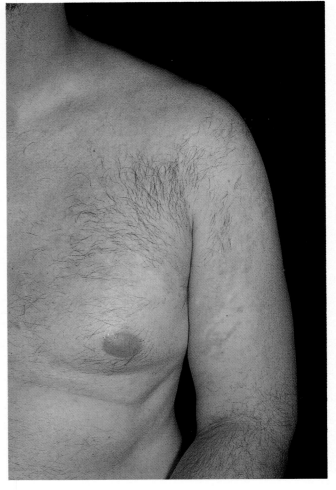

2.8
Becker's nevus. Tan patch with hypertrichosis. This is an acquired lesion that usually appears during adolescence and is much more common in males.

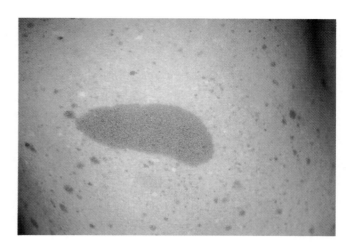

2.9
Café au lait spot in neurofibromatosis.

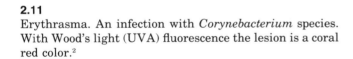

2.10
Albright's syndrome consists of a melanotic patch with an irregular border, polyostotic fibrous dysplasia of the bone, endocrine dysfunction, and precocious puberty. The café au lait macules tend to be unilateral and large in this condition.

2.11
Erythrasma. An infection with *Corynebacterium* species. With Wood's light (UVA) fluorescence the lesion is a coral red color.[2]

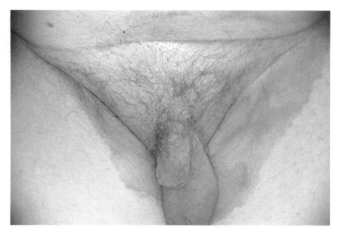

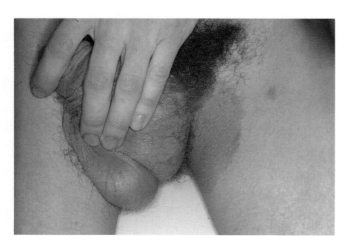

2.12
Tinea cruris. This red-tan patch has a slight scale along the border.

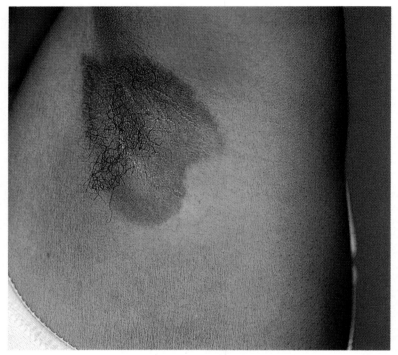

2.13
Postinflammatory hyperpigmentation due to allergic contact dermatitis.

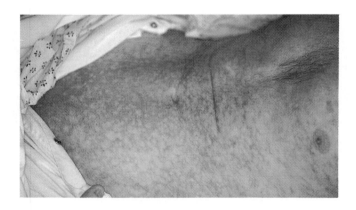

2.14
Dyskeratosis congenita. Reticulated hyperpigmented macules are present in this patient. This condition is characterized by nail dystrophy and oral leukoplakia, followed by reticulated poikiloderma that results in hyperpigmentation. These patients have an increased risk of squamous cell carcinoma.

2.15
Fixed drug eruption due to a laxative containing phenolphthalein. Note the erythematous border surrounding the brown macule.

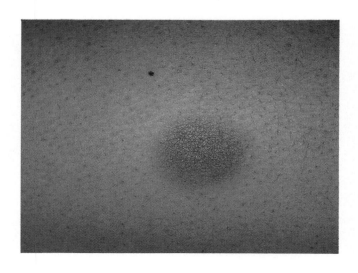

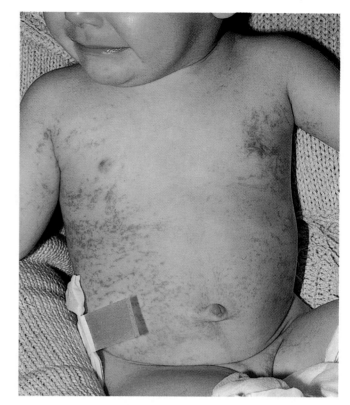

2.16
Incontinentia pigmenti. This is the third stage of this X-linked, dominantly inherited cutaneous disease. The first stage is vesicular, the second is verrucous, and the third is represented by this swirled hyperpigmentation.

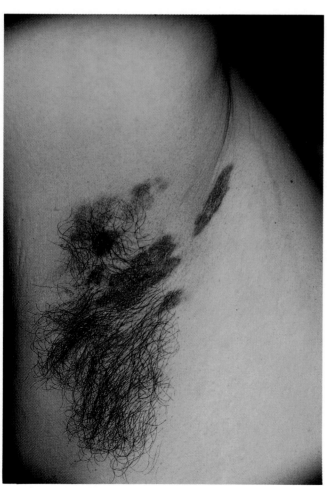

2.17
Lichen planus with an "inverse" distribution. Little or no scale or epidermal change is present.

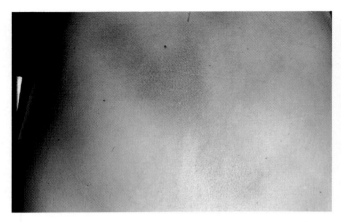

2.18
Macular amyloidosis. This condition is unrelated to any systemic disease and is localized to the skin.

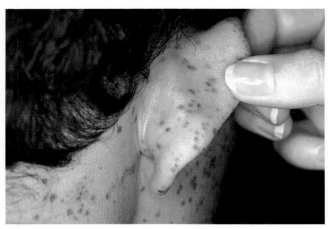

2.20
Hereditary generalized lentigines.

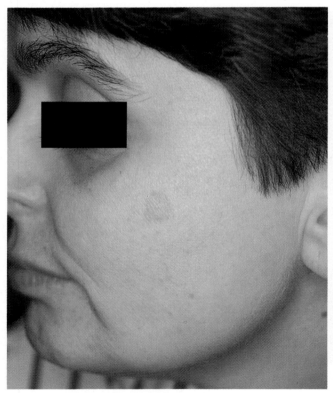

2.19
Lentigo. This is a sun-induced lesion but it may also occur on less exposed areas of the body.

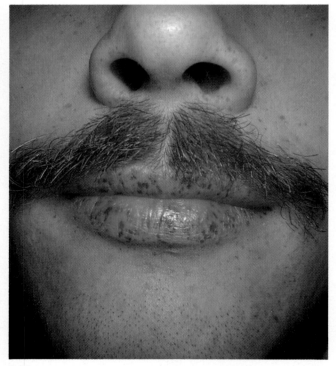

2.21
Peutz-Jeghers syndrome with brown mucosal macules. This autosomal dominant disorder combines the mucosal pigmented macules with hamartomatous polyps throughout the gastrointestinal tract.

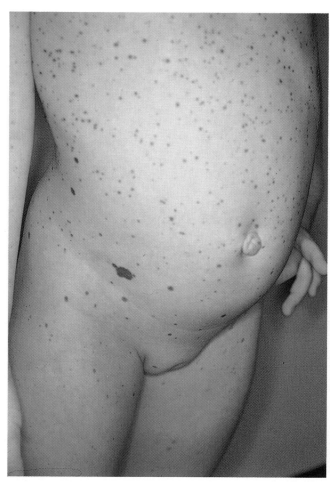

2.22
LEOPARD syndrome. This disorder combines *l*entigines, *e*lectrocardiographic abnormalities, *o*cular hypertelorism, *p*ulmonary stenosis, *a*bnormal genitalia, *r*etardation of growth, and sensorineural *d*eafness.[9]

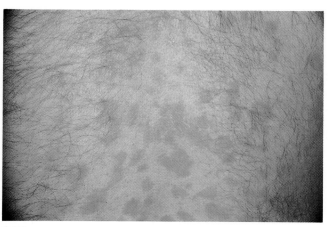

2.24
Parapsoriasis en plaque. This is an unusual appearance for this condition.

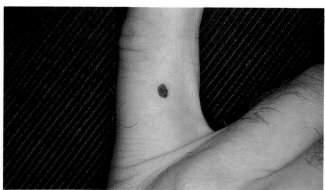

2.25
Junctional nevus.[3]

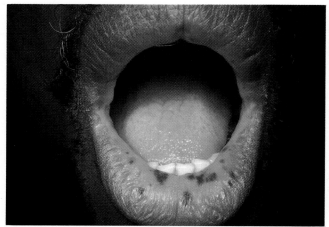

2.23
Acquired mucosal melanotic macules in an HIV-infected patient.

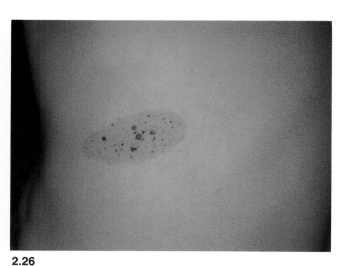

2.26
Nevus spilus. A tan patch with multiple small, darker-pigmented macules within the lesion.

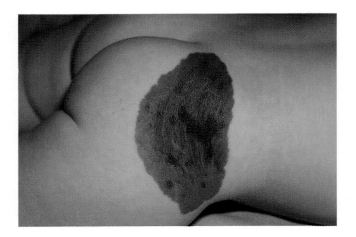

2.27
Congenital hairy nevus. This lesion is present at birth. It is distinguished from nevus spilus, which is characterized by tiny, darkly hyperpigmented macules on a lightly hyperpigmented patch and does not have hair, and Becker's nevus, which has much more hair and begins in adolescence.

2.28
Multiple architecturally atypical melanocytic macules (formerly termed dysplastic nevi).

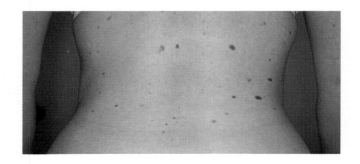

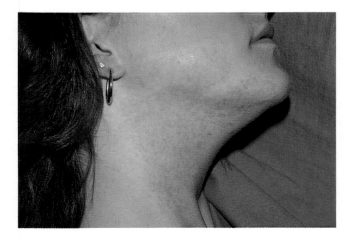

2.29
Segmental lentiginous nevus.[5]

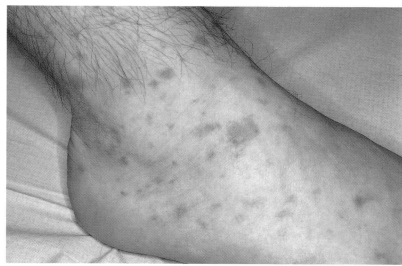

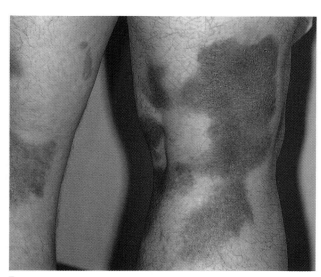

2.30

A, Capillaritis (progressive pigmentary purpura). This nonblanchable eruption may have hyperpigmented macules as its only manifestation. Note that in this case purpura is absent. B, Capillaritis with a deeper brown color.

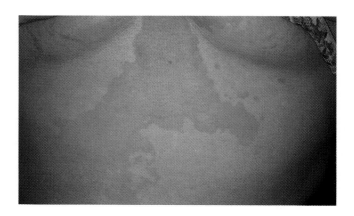

2.31

Tinea versicolor. This process rarely has clinically appreciable scale, yet light scraping shows abundant epidermal debris to be present.

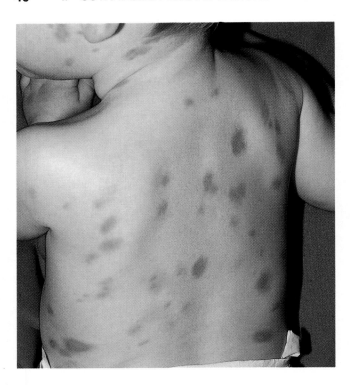

2.32
Urticaria pigmentosa. These patients have multiple hyperpigmented macules that release histamine and lead to urtication when stroked (Darier's sign).

Brown Macules Primarily on the Palms and/or Soles

Similar lesions may occur on other body surfaces, with the exception of tinea nigra palmaris and talon noir.

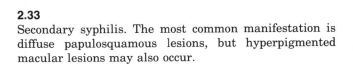

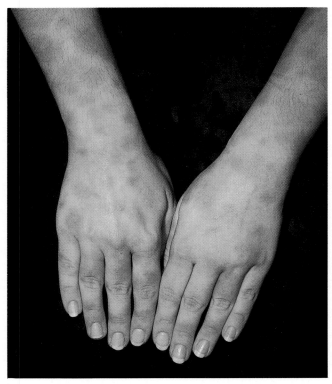

2.33
Secondary syphilis. The most common manifestation is diffuse papulosquamous lesions, but hyperpigmented macular lesions may also occur.

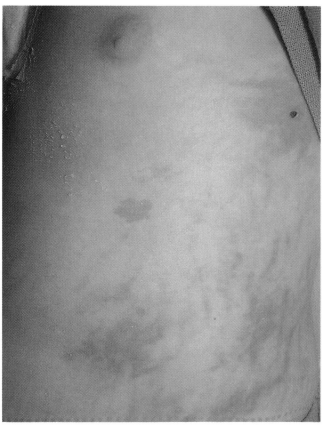

2.34
Drug-induced hyperpigmentation. Bleomycin tends to induce a streaky hyperpigmentation within areas of previous, even minor, injury to the skin.

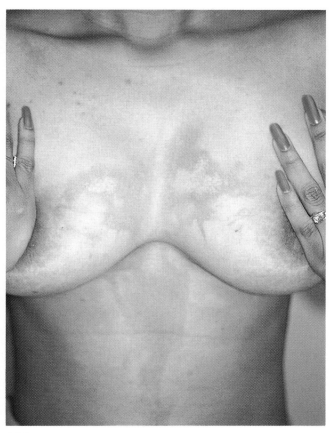

2.36
This patient's hyperpigmentation followed a burn from an accidental spill of coffee.

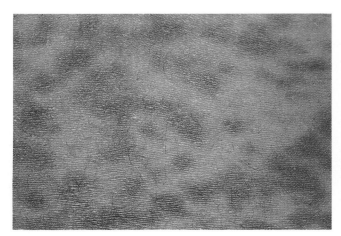

2.35
Darkly pigmented skin may have profound residual hyperpigmentation after a drug eruption.

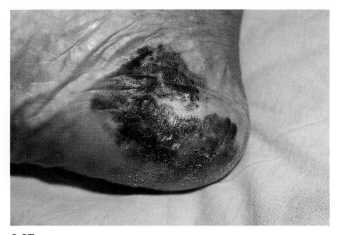

2.37
Acrolentiginous melanoma. This brown-to-black flat lesion has irregular borders and variable pigmentation.

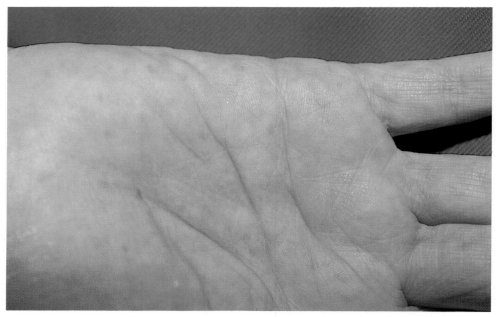

2.38
Cronkhite-Canada syndrome. Characterized by tan macules that may be generalized, gastrointestinal polyps with diarrhea, abdominal pain, malabsorption, diffuse alopecia, and nail changes.

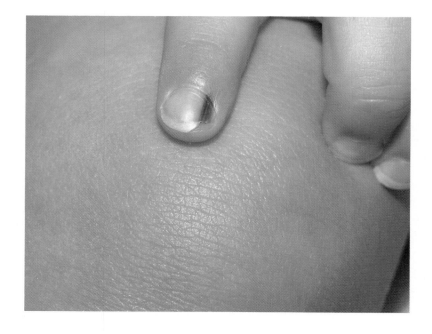

2.39
Junctional nevus of the nail bed.

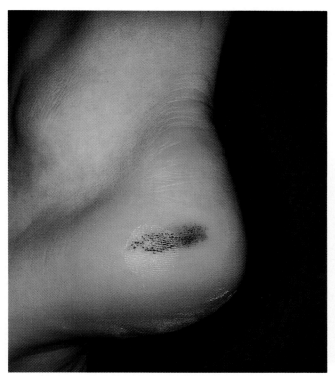

2.40
Talon noir. This brown-macular lesion is localized to the heel and is due to hemorrhage after trauma. This change is usually associated with athletic activity.

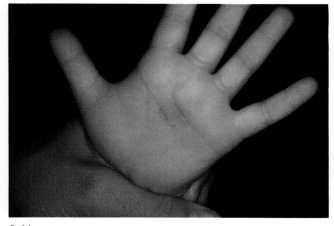

2.41
Tinea nigra palmaris is due to a dematiaceous fungus known currently as *Exophilia werneckii*.

Diffuse Brown Hyperpigmentation (Table I)

TABLE I Differential Diagnosis of Diffuse (Generalized) Hyperpigmentation
ACTH- or MSH-producing tumors (e.g., oat cell carcinoma of lung)* Addison's disease Arsenic ingestion Drug induced (antimalarials, some cytotoxic agents) Hemochromatosis ("bronze" diabetes) Malabsorption syndrome (Whipple's disease, celiac sprue) Melanoma Melanotropic hormone injection* Pheochromocytoma Porphyrias (porphyria cutanea tarda, variegate porphyria) Pregnancy Progressive systemic sclerosis and related conditions PUVA (psoralen plus ultraviolet A) therapy for psoriasis, vitiligo*

*Accentuation on sun-exposed surfaces.

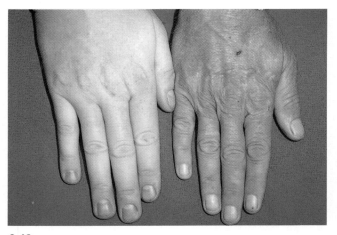

2.42
Addison's disease. The abnormal hand is seen on the right and is uniformly hyperpigmented.

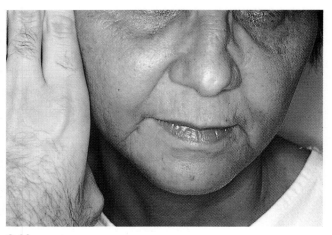

2.44
Hemochromatosis, also known as "bronze diabetes," combines diabetes mellitus, cirrhosis, and generalized hyperpigmentation. These patients have iron overload.

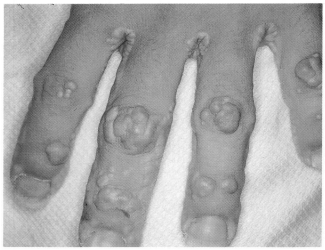

2.43
Primary biliary cirrhosis. This patient has had tuberous and eruptive xanthomas on a diffusely hyperpigmented background.

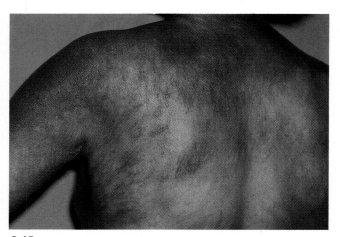

2.45
Scleroderma. Occasionally, patients will develop a diffuse hyperpigmentation.

Generalized Congenital

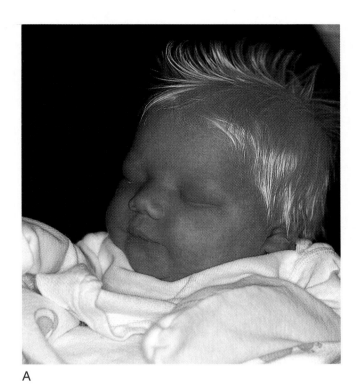

A

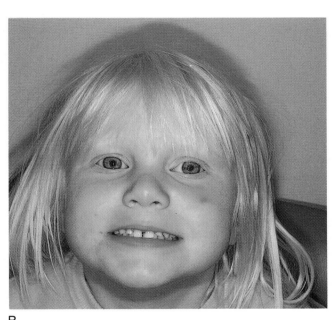

B

2.46
Albinism. *A*, Diffuse and total pigment loss in the hair. *B*, Diffuse and total pigment loss.

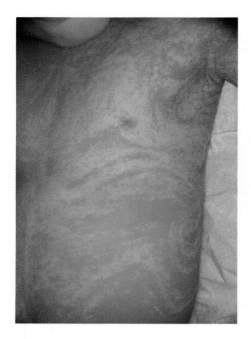

2.47
Hypomelanosis of Ito (or incontinentia pigmenti achromians). An inherited neurocutaneous disorder, perhaps inherited in an autosomal dominant fashion, and characterized by linear streaks and whorls of hypopigmentation as seen. It can be distinguished from incontinentia pigmenti, which usually has vesicular, verrucous, and hyperpigmented phases before hypopigmentation.

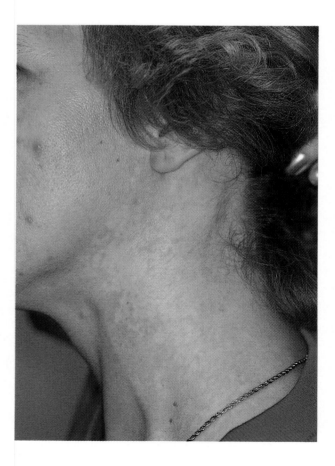

2.48
Nevus depigmentosus. An uncommon, perhaps nevoid leukoderma characterized by irregular, feathered, or serrated margins. The lesion is almost always unilateral.

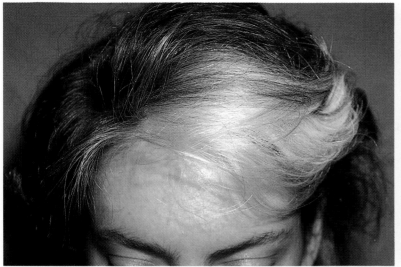

2.49

A, B, Piebaldism. A congenital leukoderma characterized by a white forelock *(A)* and hyperpigmented macules within an amelanotic patch surrounded by normally pigmented skin *(B).* The general health of these patients is not affected. The inheritance pattern is autosomal dominant.

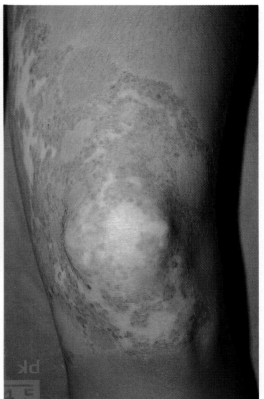

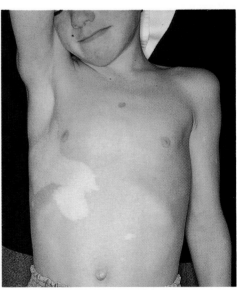

B

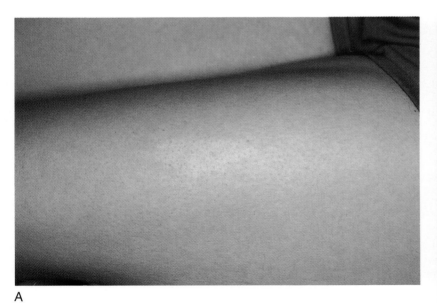

2.50

A, B, Tuberous sclerosis. A typical small ash-leaf macule *(A)* and a large, irregular, hypopigmented macule *(B)* are among the leukodermatous manifestations of this condition. This is a neurocutaneous disorder (phakomatosis) characterized by multiple hamartomatous tumors that commonly may affect the central nervous system, kidneys, heart, eyes, and skin. It is inherited in an autosomal dominant pattern, but many cases are sporadic mutations.

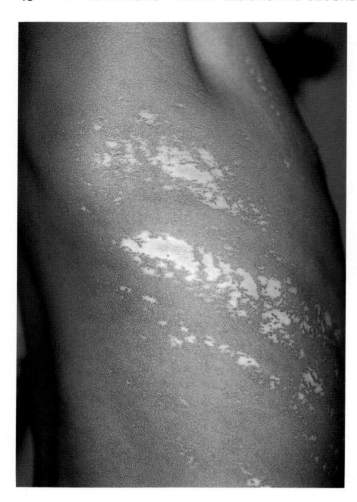

2.51
Focal dermal hypoplasia (Goltz's syndrome) is characterized by atrophy and linear hyper- or hypopigmented skin.[2]

Acquired

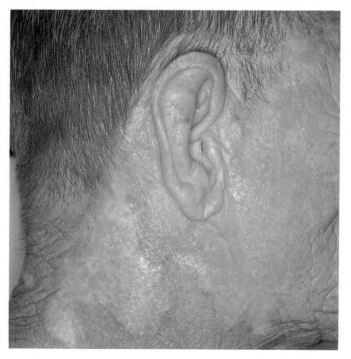

2.52
Chronic cutaneous lupus erythematosus can lead to hypopigmentation. This man has erythema from sun exposure of his hypopigmented skin.[2]

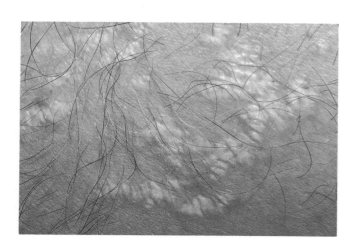

2.53
Halo nevi. Gradual lightening of the skin occurs surrounding a nevus. Eventually the entire pigmented surface can disappear.[5]

2.54
Lichen sclerosus et atrophicus. A hypopigmented patch with epidermal atrophy and perhaps some slight scale. This condition frequently has small pits, known as dells, which can be seen in this example.

2.55
Degos disease. This condition is due to localized vascular infarction. The result is small, ivory white atrophic lesions. These patients also have vascular problems of the central nervous system and gastrointestinal tract.

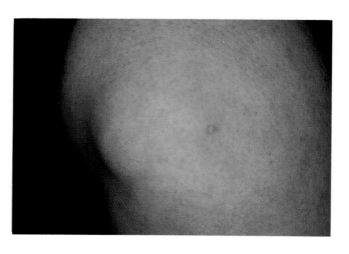

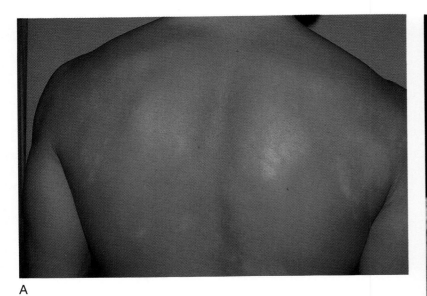

A

2.56
A, B, Pityriasis alba. A hypopigmented, mild form of atopic eczema.

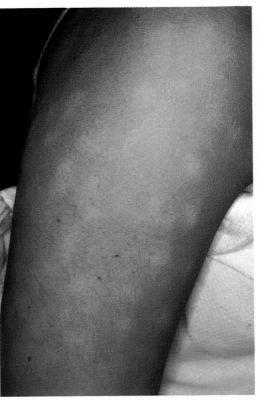

B

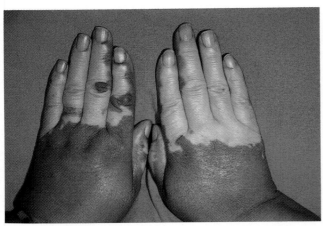

2.57
Phenolic depigmentation. Chemically induced depigmentation that simulates vitiligo.

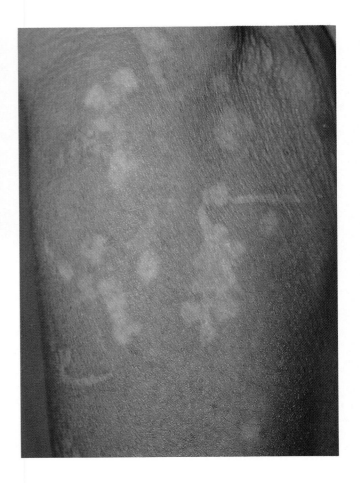

2.58
Hypomelanosis after physical trauma in a patient with neurotic excoriations.

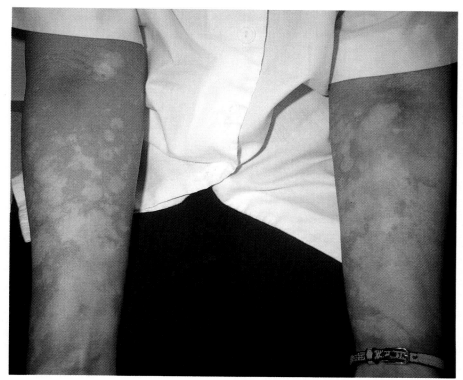

2.59
Postinflammatory hypopigmentation in a patient with atopic eczema.

2.60
Idiopathic guttate hypomelanosis. Small hypopigmented
macules on the anterior shins.

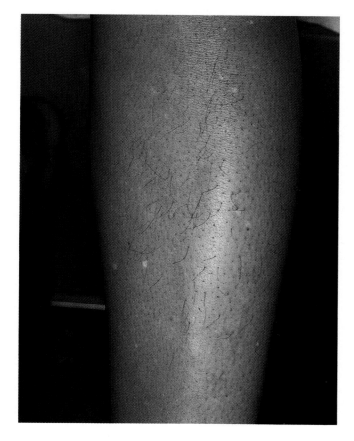

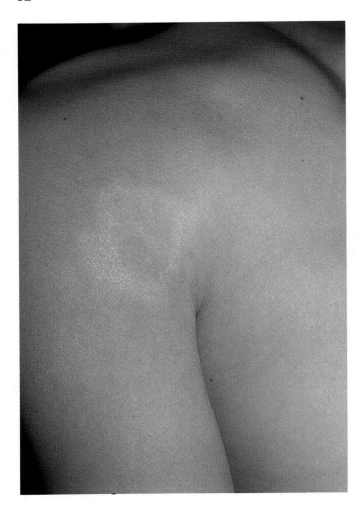

2.61
Hypopigmented anesthetic macule of tuberculous leprosy.

2.62
Sarcoidosis. Hypopigmentation surrounds the erythematous papules in this patient.

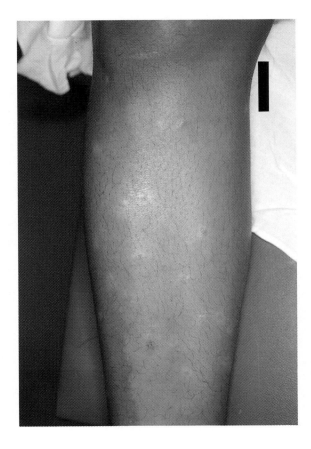

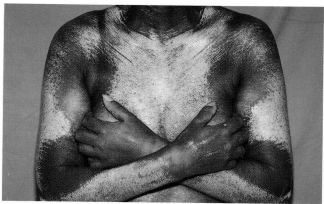

2.63
Progressive systemic sclerosis (scleroderma) frequently manifests as a leukoderma in which there is perifollicular retention of pigment.

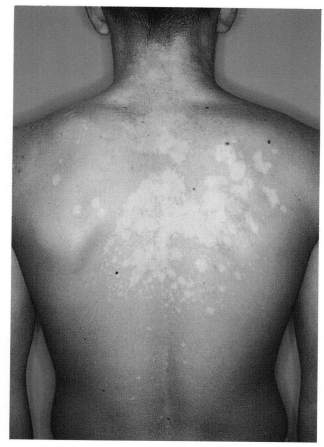

2.65
Tinea versicolor. Hypopigmented patches with fine scale are seen.

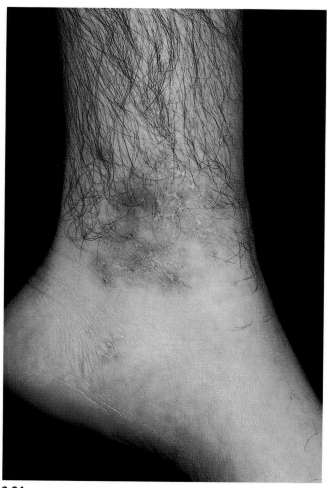

2.64
Atrophie blanche is a disease of vascular insufficiency in which there is reticulated purpura and ulcerations. The ulcerations heal with stellate white (ivory) scars.

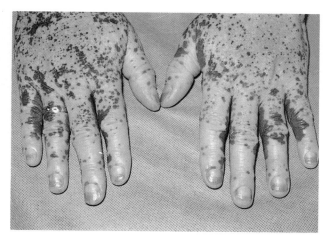

2.66
Vitiligo.

BLUE MACULES

Congenital

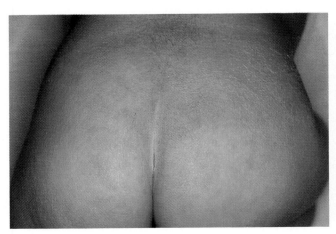

2.67
Mongolian spot or congenital dermal melanocytosis, commonly observed in African-Americans and Asians at birth.[2]

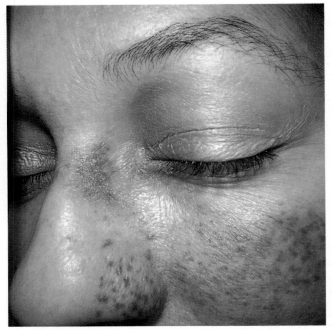

2.68
Nevus of Ota (oculodermal melanocytosis).

Acquired

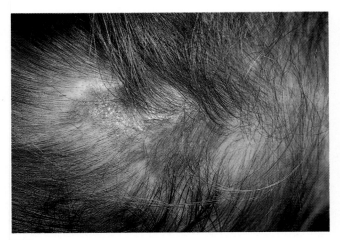

2.69
Blue nevus: plaque form. More commonly these lesions are small nodules.

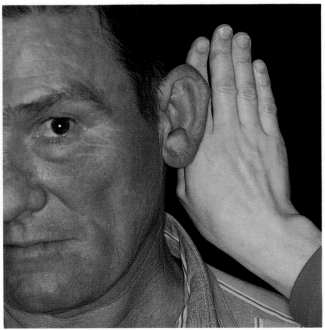

2.70
Amiodarone pigmentation. This change is photodistributed.

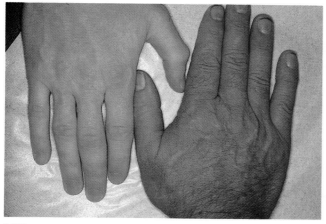

2.71
Argyria. This slate-gray color is generalized. The normal hand is on the left.

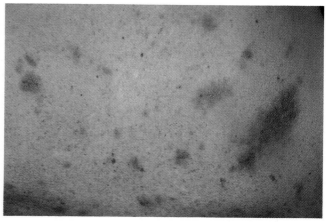

2.73
HIV-associated Kaposi's sarcoma can be macular.

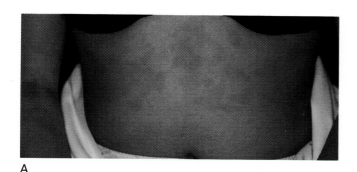

A

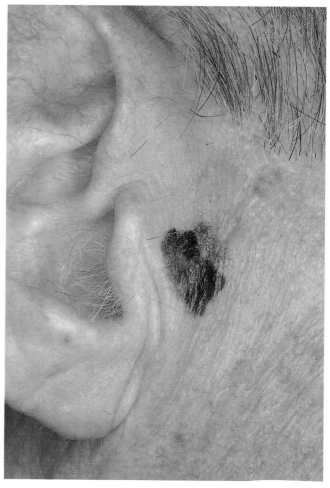

B

2.72
A, Erythema dyschromicum perstans (ashy dermatosis) is an idiopathic condition that may follow a subtle inflammatory dermatosis. B, Erythema dyschromicum perstans in a Cuban woman.[2]

2.74
Lentigo maligna melanoma. A blue-black pigmented lesion on the face. This type of melanoma has a prolonged horizontal growth phase and thus is macular for long periods.[8]

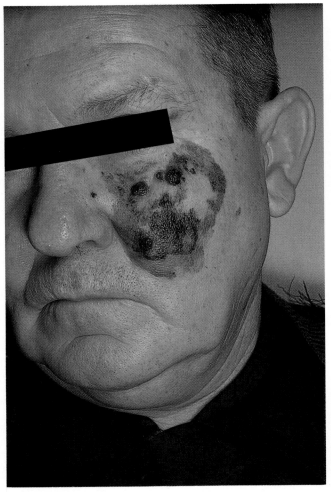

2.75
Lentigo maligna melanoma with evidence of regression.

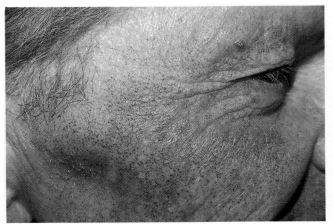

2.76
Ochronosis. An inborn error of metabolism in which homogentisic acid oxidase is absent, inherited in an autosomal recessive manner and characterized by cutaneous pigmentation, dark urine, and arthritis.[12]

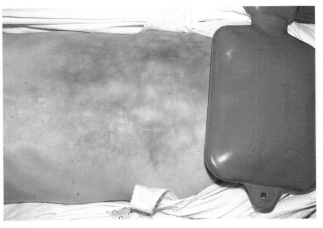

2.77
Erythema ab igne. This case was due to repeated use of a hot water bottle. This patient has a reticulated gray-blue pigmentation.

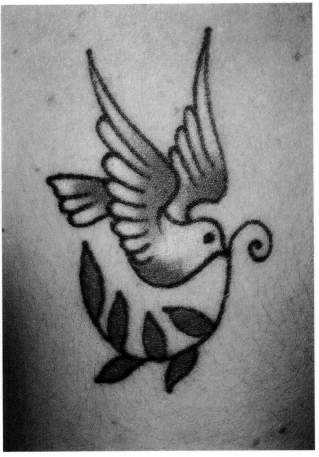

2.78
Tattoo. An intentional instillation of foreign material.

RED MACULAR LESIONS

Red macules can be divided into transient lesions (e.g., flushing), exanthems, vascular lesions, or scattered inflammatory lesions. Flushing occurs in the carcinoid syndrome, mast cell disease, pheochromocytomas, central nervous system disease, and acne rosacea. Telangiectasias (see also Chapter 8) and reticulated erythemas (see also Chapters 7 and 8), while often macular, are also described in other sections.

Viral exanthems and drug eruptions are frequently described as a "diffuse maculopapular" rash. In fact many of these instances are a diffuse confluence of erythematous macules. Many of these eruptions are clinically indistinct without the benefit of the history, other physical findings, and laboratory evaluation. Thus, only a few examples of these conditions are shown.

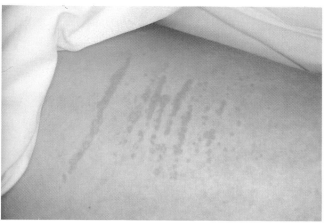

2.79
Juvenile rheumatoid arthritis is characterized by fever, arthritis, and evanescent erythema. Occasionally, urticarial lesions are also present.

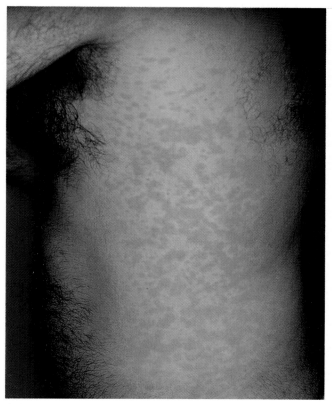

2.80
Viral exanthem due to a presumed enterovirus infection.

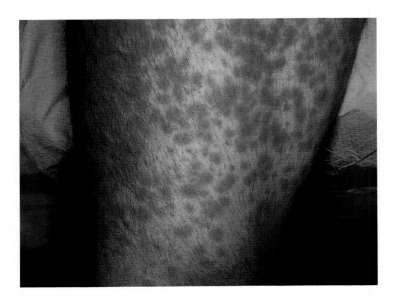

2.81
Dusky erythema is seen in this patient with infectious mononucleosis who had been given ampicillin.

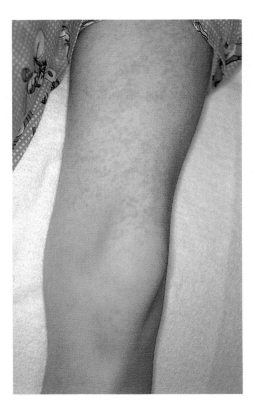

2.82
Kawasaki's disease (mucocutaneous lymph node syndrome) is associated with a variety of cutaneous eruptions. This patient had confluent erythematous macules. Erythema multiforme and perineal dusky erythema with scaling are other common skin changes. Patients also have fever, lymphadenopathy, peripheral edema, and mucosal involvement. Palmoplantar desquamation is quite common. These patients may develop coronary artery aneurysms.

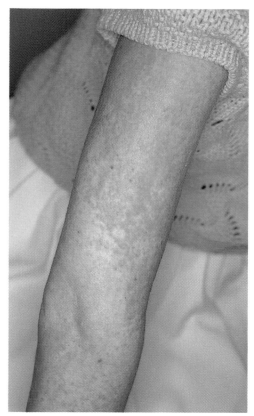

2.83
Drug eruption. Confluent macular erythema due to ingestion of a nonsteroidal anti-inflammatory agent.

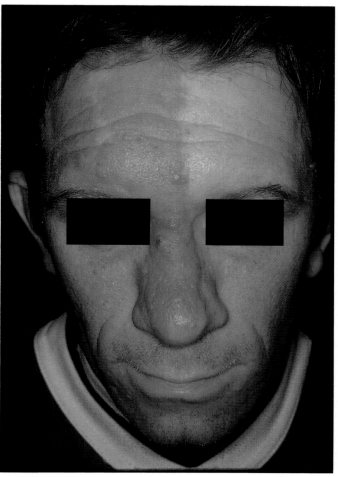

2.85
Nevus flammeus in the Sturge-Weber syndrome (encephalotrigeminal angiomatosis). A sporadic disorder in which the angiomatous lesions affect the skin, eye, and central nervous system.

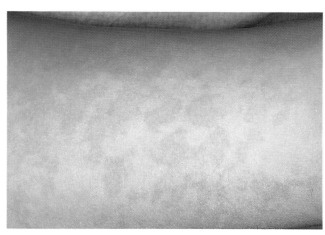

2.84
Fifth disease (erythema infectiosum) is a parvovirus infection.

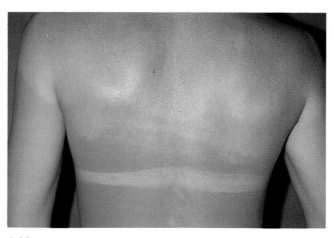

2.86
Sunburn reaction. Note that the areas covered with clothing and the upper back, on which a sunscreen was applied, are not affected.[2]

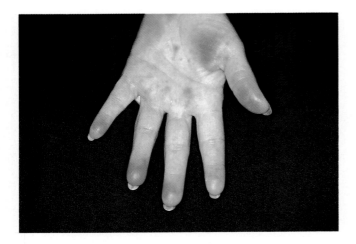

2.87
Acral erythema of chemotherapy. In this case methotrexate was believed to be the cause.

2.88
Inflammatory metastatic carcinoma of the breast.

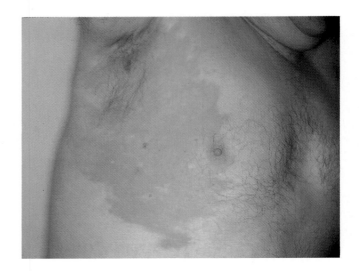

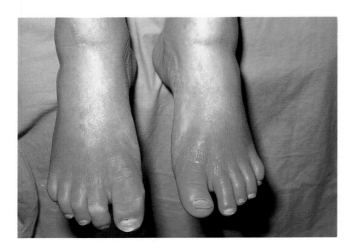

2.89
Erythromelalgia. A rare disorder characterized by painful acral erythema that is relieved by cooling.

3

PAPULAR LESIONS AND PLAQUES

Papules are raised lesions that are usually less than 0.5 cm in diameter and about as elevated as they are wide. Plaques are lesions in which the diameter of the lesion is greater than its height, forming plateau-like lesions. Papules and plaques can be inflammatory or neoplastic. This category of lesions can be distinguished by color (skin tone, red, brown, blue-black, yellow), by whether there is a surface change such as scale (papulosquamous disorders), by configuration (linear), or by symptoms (pain, see Table II).

TABLE II
Painful Papulonodular Lesions

Angiolipoma
Chondrodermatitis nodularis helicis
Eccrine spiradenoma
Glomus tumor
Leiomyoma
Neuroma

FLESH-COLORED PAPULES

These lesions may have pigmentation similar to that observed in the surrounding skin.

Pedunculated Flesh-Colored Papules

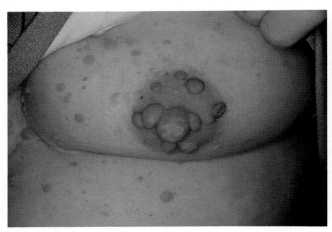

3.1
Multiple neurofibromas are present in this patient with neurofibromatosis.

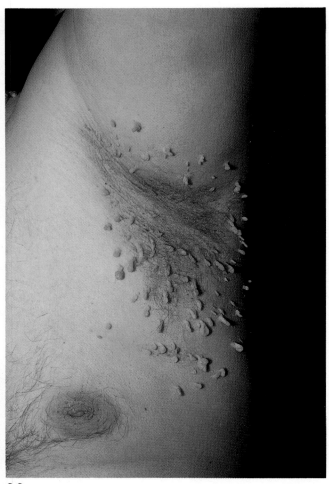

3.3
Multiple skin tags are present in this obese man, who also has pseudoacanthosis nigricans.

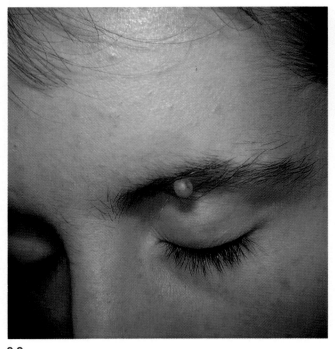

3.2
Intradermal nevi are often elevated and may be nonpigmented.

3.4
Digital fibroepithelial papilloma. A rare, pedunculated tumor.

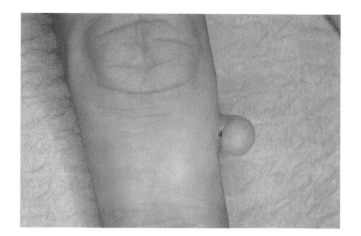

Scattered Flesh-Colored Papules

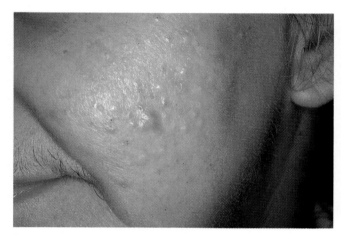

3.5
Multiple closed comedones in acne.[2]

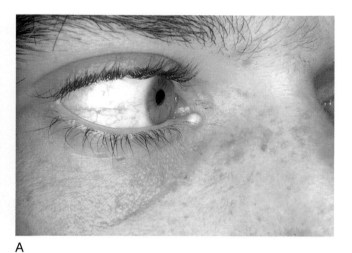

A

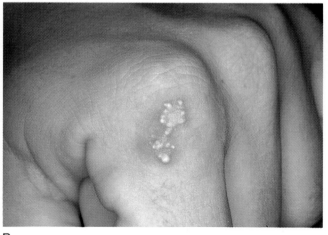

B

3.7
A, Milial cyst. A small, epidermal inclusion cyst. B, Multiple milial cysts after an injury to the skin with re-epithelialization.

3.6
Giant comedo. This flesh-colored lesion has a central expressible core.

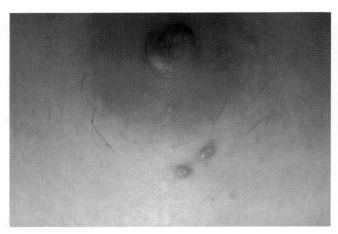

3.8
Molluscum contagiosum. Small papules with a central umbilication.

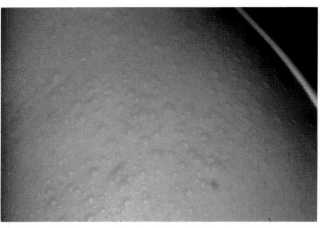

3.10
Lichen planus (shoulder). Although usually pigmented or erythematous, this can at times be flesh-colored. Also, there is no surface change in this patient.

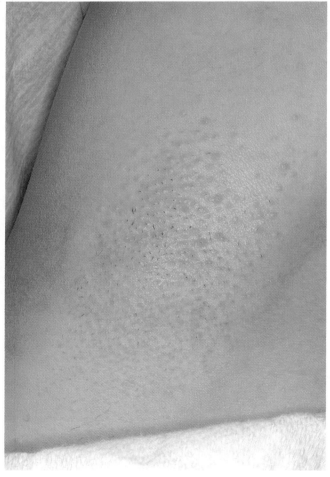

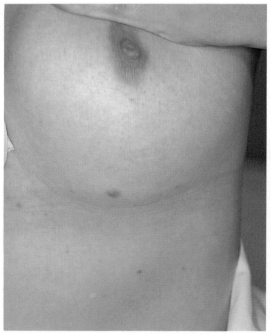

3.11
Accessory nipple. A papular lesion the same color as the skin of the nipple. These lesions occur along the "nipple" line.

3.9
Apocrine miliaria (Fox-Fordyce disease).

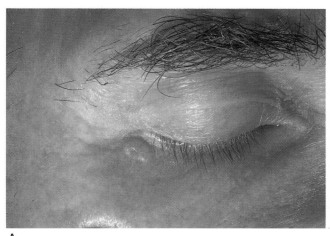

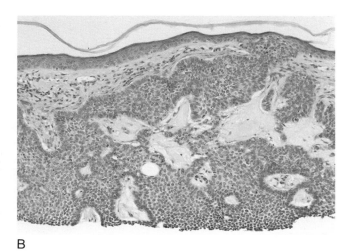

A

B

3.12
A, Basal cell epithelioma. A small translucent papule along the lower lid near the inner canthus. *B*, Histopathologic changes of basal cell epithelioma.

3.13
Condylomata acuminata (genital warts). Flesh-colored papules are present at the urethral meatus and along the shaft of the penis.

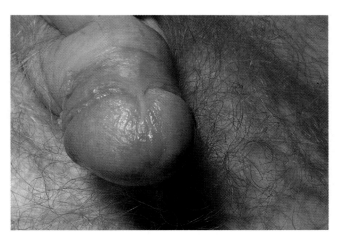

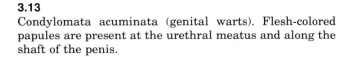

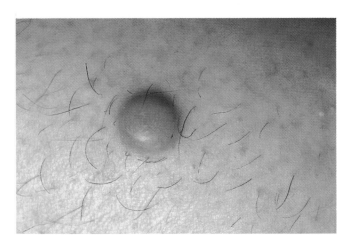

3.14
Dermatofibroma.

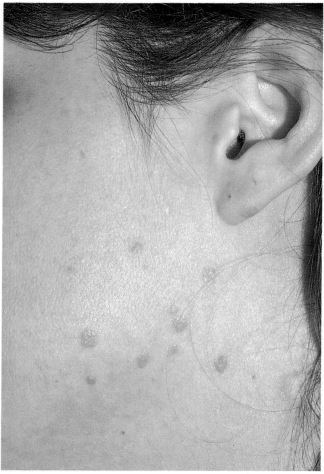

3.15
Flat warts.

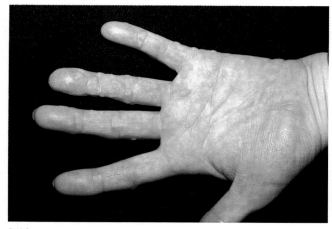

3.16
Verruca vulgaris (common viral warts). These papules often have verrucous surface changes.

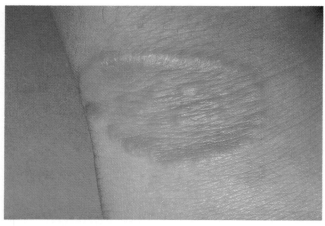

3.17
Granuloma annulare. An active border with a dermal infiltrative process. No surface change is noted.

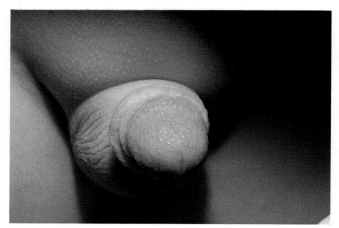

3.18
Lichen nitidus. Multiple minute, flesh-colored papules.

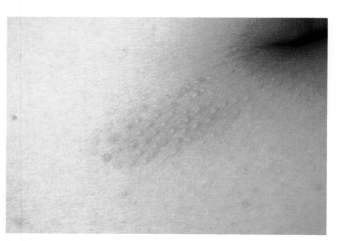

3.19
Lichen spinulosus.

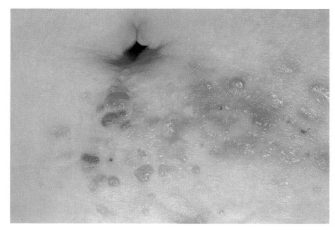

3.20
Periumbilical lesions of lymphangioma circumscriptum. Some of the lesions contain blood, but most are flesh-colored or translucent papules.

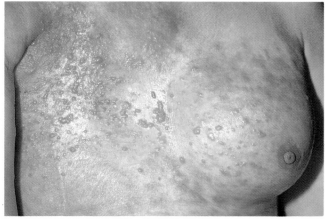

3.21
Metastatic breast carcinoma. Some lesions are flesh-colored; others are red from surrounding inflammation.

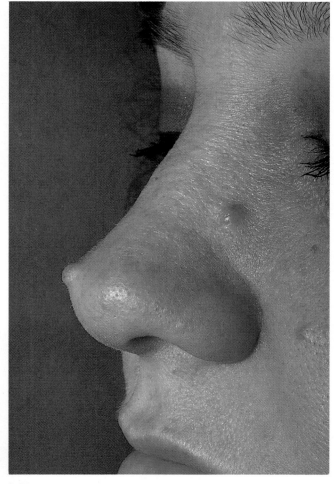

3.22
Intradermal nevus, nonpedunculated.

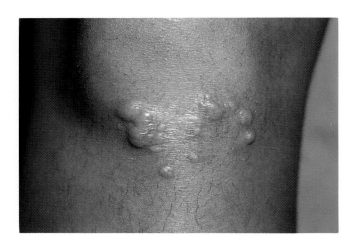

3.23
Sarcoidosis. Multiple dermal papular lesions on the knee.

Facial Flesh-Colored Papules

The following lesions are found primarily on the face but may also occur elsewhere.

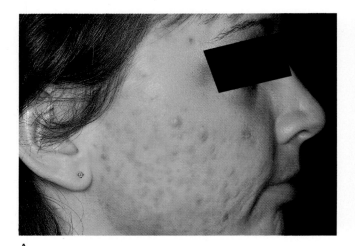

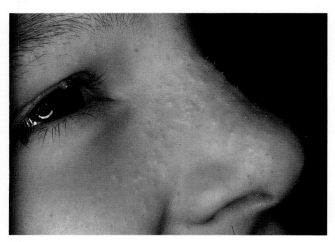

A   B

3.24
A, Acne vulgaris. Flesh-colored papules with some erythematous nodules and cysts. *B*, Comedonal acne in a preadolescent boy.

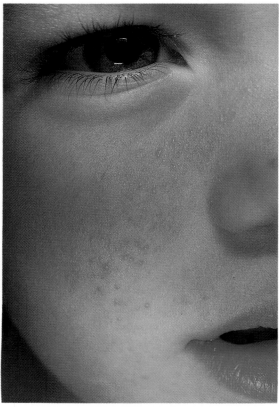

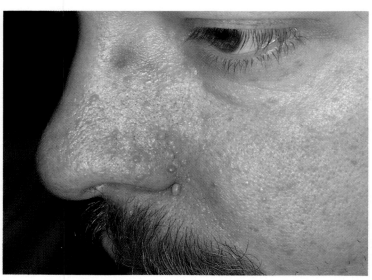

B

3.25
A, Adenoma sebaceum of tuberous sclerosis. Early lesions: flesh-colored and erythematous papules. These lesions are histopathologically angiofibromas. *B*, Later in life the lesions of tuberous sclerosis may enlarge.

A

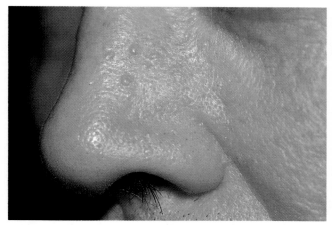

3.26
Basal cell nevus syndrome. An autosomal dominant disorder. Each of the flesh-colored papules in this patient was a basal cell carcinoma.[5]

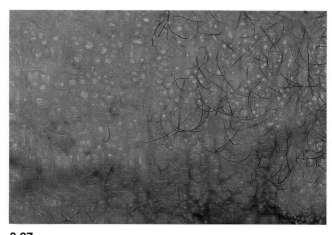

3.27
Colloid milium. These flesh-colored papules are due to infiltration of colloid in the dermis. This material is similar to amyloid histopathologically.

3.28
Cowden's disease (multiple hamartoma syndrome). Multiple tricholemmomas on the central face. This autosomal dominant disorder is characterized by tricholemmomas, mucosal papillomas, thyroid tumors, breast tumors, and hamartomatous gastrointestinal polyps.

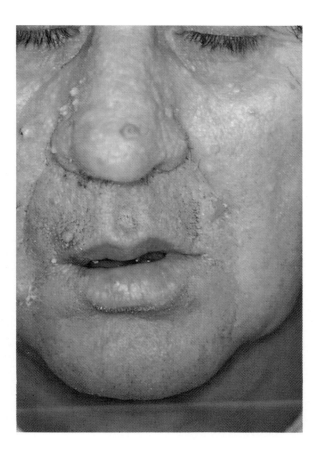

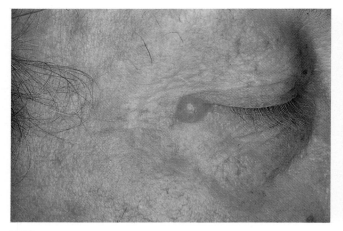

3.29
Eccrine hidrocystoma of the lateral canthus.

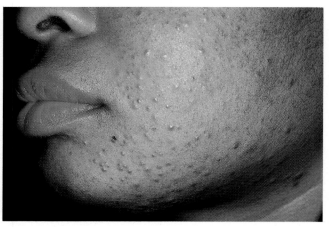

3.32
Sarcoidosis. Acneiform lesions.[3]

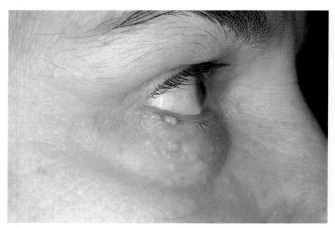

3.30
Apocrine hidrocystoma along the lid margin and multiple syringomas on the lower eyelid.[3]

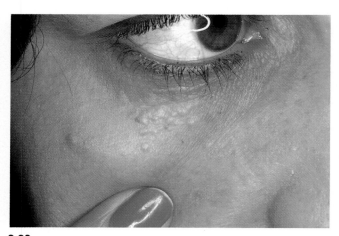

3.33
Multiple syringomas on the lower eyelid.[3]

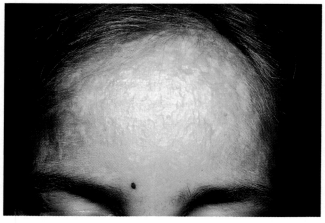

3.31
Lipoid proteinosis. Dermal infiltrate of hyaline material.

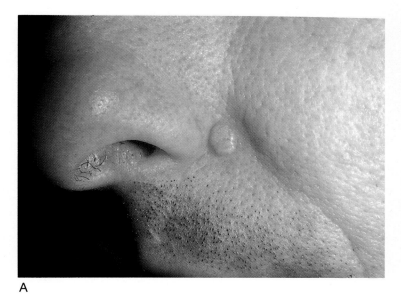

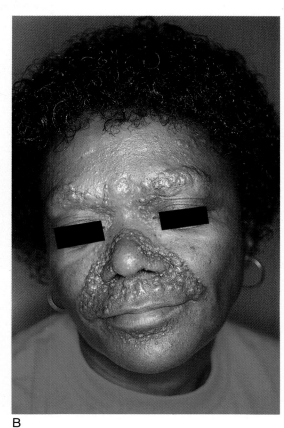

A

B

3.34
A, Trichoepithelioma, which is often clinically indistinguishable from a basal cell carcinoma.
B, Multiple trichoepitheliomas, which may clinically simulate the adenoma sebaceum lesions of tuberous sclerosis.

3.35
Sebaceous gland hyperplasia. Flesh-colored or white-yellow papules.[5]

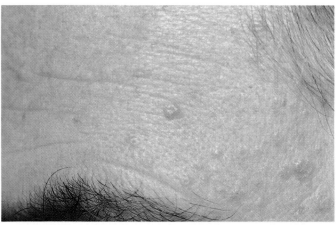

Other Flesh-Colored Papules and Plaques

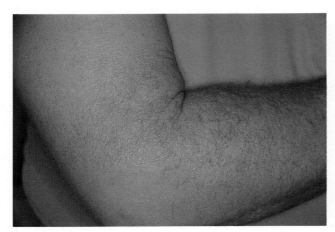

3.36
Colloid milium.[2]

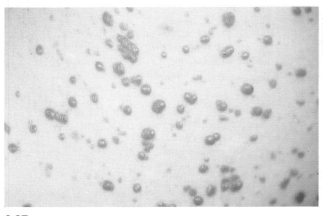

3.37
Xanthoma disseminatum. Slightly pink papules representing an infiltrate filled with lipid-laden histiocytes.

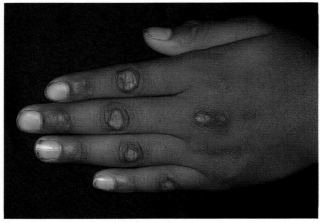

3.38
Knuckle pads (thickened plaques over the knuckles).

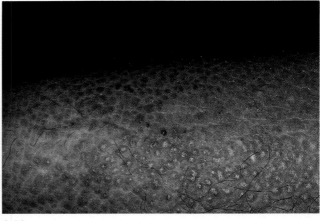

3.39
Lichen amyloidosus. Infiltrate of amyloid, a proteinaceous material, in the skin. This is a local process unassociated with systemic disease.

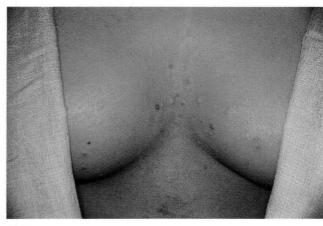

3.40
Steatocystoma multiplex. Multiple small cysts lined by epithelium plus sebaceous glands.

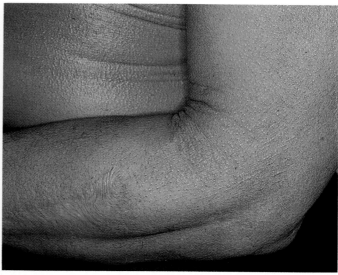

B

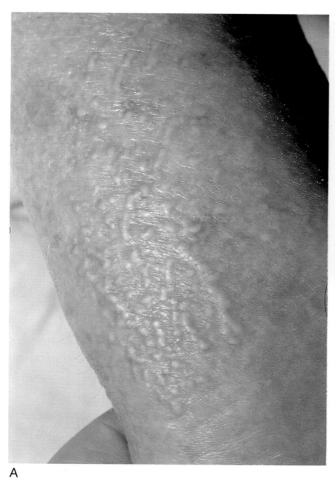

A

3.41

A, Papular mucinosis (lichen myxedematosus). Dermal infiltrate of mucin. These patients frequently have a mono-clonal paraprotein but rarely develop multiple myeloma. The lesions often have a linear array. *B,* Papular mucinosis in a black patient.

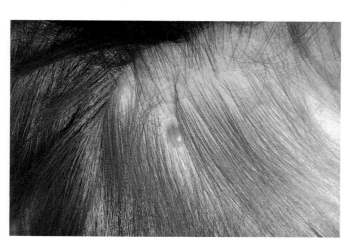

3.42

Juvenile xanthogranuloma. Slightly red-yellow papule in a child.

ERYTHEMATOUS PAPULES AND PLAQUES

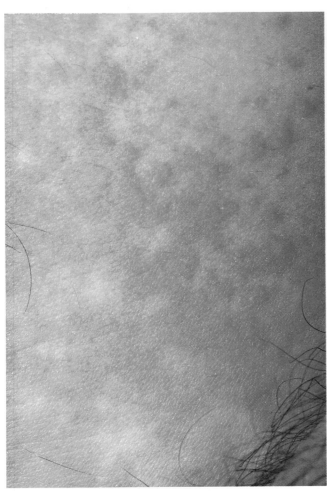

3.43
Cholinergic urticaria. These small, urticarial, slightly erythematous papules appear after exercising or becoming overheated.

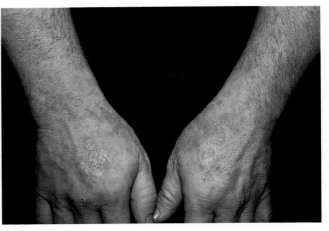

3.44
Contact dermatitis can begin as small red papules and plaques. This patient's condition was due to epoxy resin hypersensitivity.

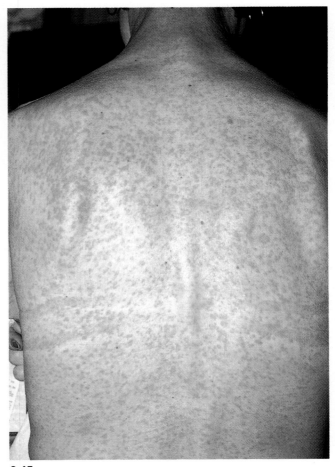

3.45
Drug eruptions can be represented by multiple erythematous papules. This one was due to phenobarbital. The lesions may coalesce to form plaques.

3.46
Erythema multiforme. Erythematous urticarial papules and plaques with central vesiculation. The most common causes of this condition are drugs and infections. Herpes simplex virus infection is perhaps the most common cause of recurrent erythema multiforme.

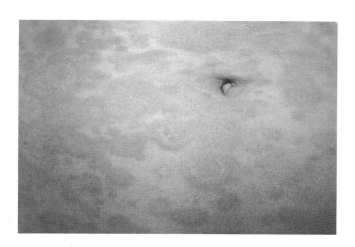

3.47
Pityriasis rosea. An acute, self-limited eruption characterized by salmon-colored plaques with a fine scale just inside the margin (collarette of scale).

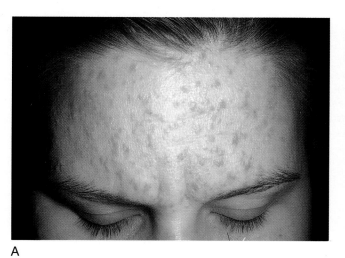

A

B

3.48
A, B, Polymorphous light eruption. Erythematous papules that may become confluent and form plaques. This eruption occurs in a photosensitive distribution (B).

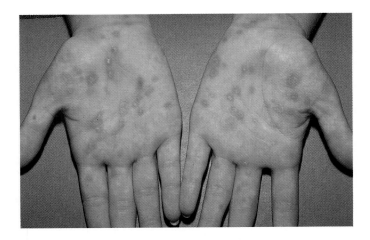

3.49
Secondary syphilis. Erythematous, slightly scaly plaques on the palms. Additional lesions in this patient simulated those of pityriasis rosea.

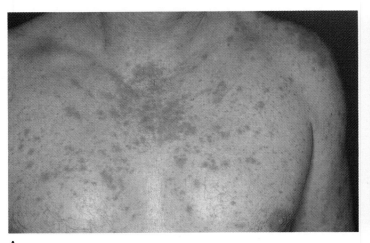

A

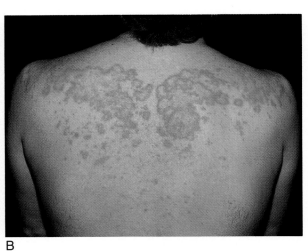

B

3.50
A to *C,* Subacute cutaneous lupus erythematosus. A nonscarring form of cutaneous lupus erythematosus, commonly associated with mild systemic disease and a variety of autoantibodies, in particular the anti-Ro (SS-A). The early lesions often mimic those of polymorphous light eruption *(A)* but progress to form annular plaques *(B)* or scaly plaques (papulosquamous lesions) *(C).*

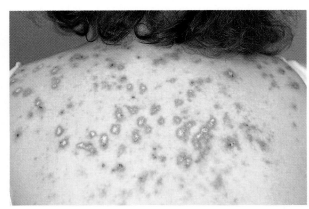

C

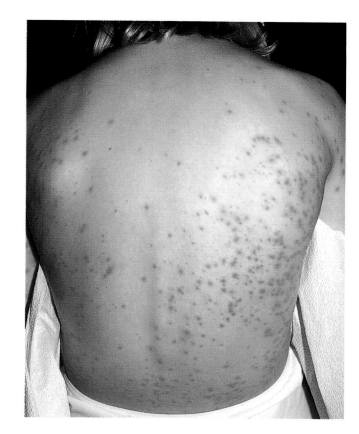

3.51
Hot tub folliculitis. Perifollicular erythematous papules and pustules due to *Pseudomonas* infection. This process is self-limited and does not require systemic antibiotics.

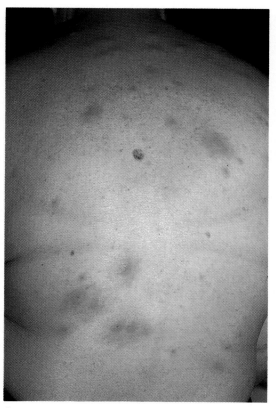

A

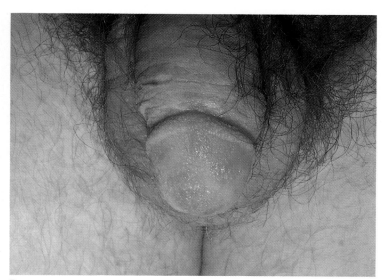

B

3.52
A, B, Insect bites result in a persistent erythematous papule or plaque. The agents in these cases were bed bugs *(A)* and scabies *(B)*.

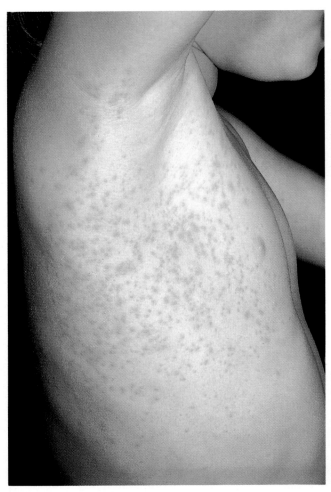

3.53
Miliaria rubra. Heat-induced eccrine sweat retention.

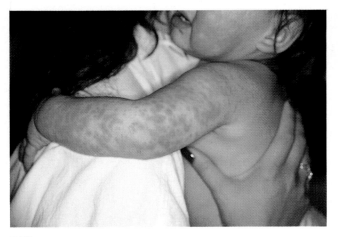

3.54
Viral exanthem. As is the case with erythematous macules, a variety of agents can cause this otherwise nonspecific eruption.[6]

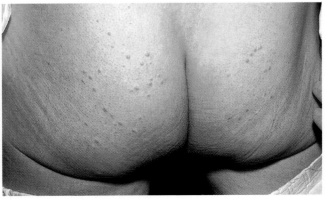

3.55
Eruptive xanthoma in a poorly controlled diabetic patient. These lesions are usually erythematous-yellow papules and are associated with hypertriglyceridemia.

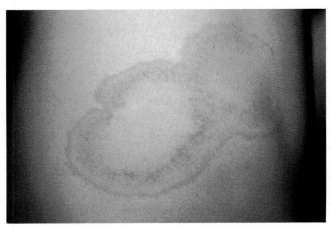

3.56
Erythema annulare centrifugum. This plaque expands gradually with a scale that "trails" behind the border. This process is a reactive dermatosis often due to a fungal infection elsewhere on the body.

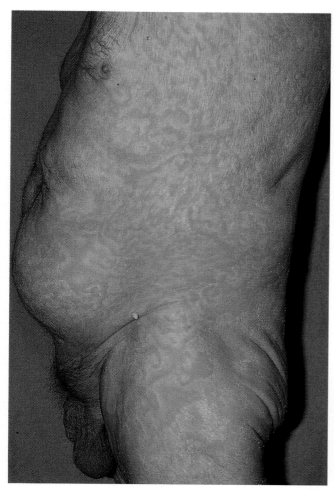

3.57
Erythema gyratum repens. These slightly scaly erythematous plaques form a bizarre "grain of wood" appearance, almost always associated with an internal neoplasm.

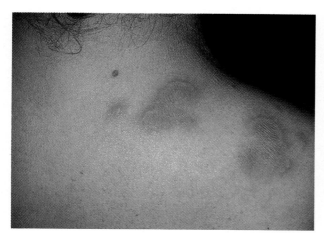

3.58
Erythema elevatum diutinum. An unusual form of leukocytoclastic vasculitis usually localized to extensor surfaces. These patients rarely have systemic manifestations.

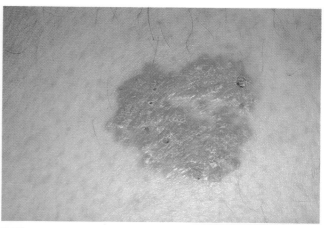

3.59
Bowen's disease. An in situ form of squamous cell carcinoma. This erythematous plaque is often mistakenly treated as eczema or psoriasis before biopsy confirmation.

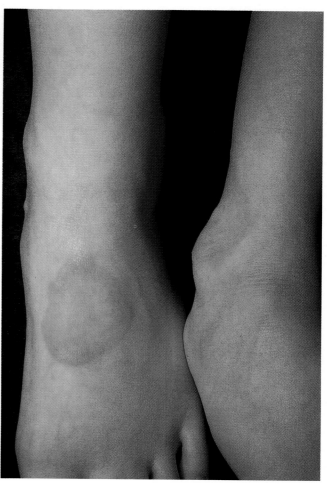

3.60
Granuloma annulare. Erythematous annular plaque.

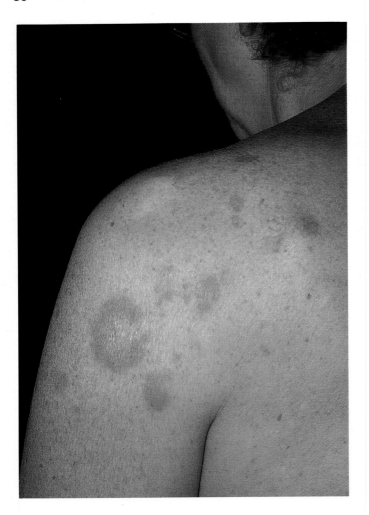

3.61
Benign lymphocytic infiltrate of the skin.

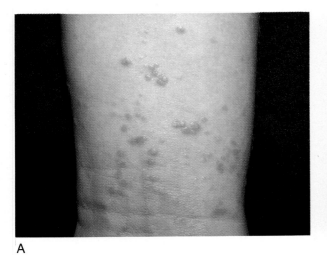

A

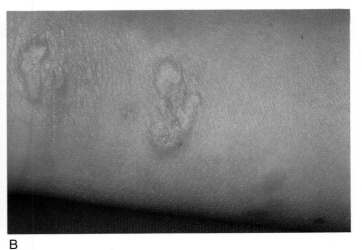

B

3.62
A, B, Lichen planus. Flat top polygonal papules and small plaques with a reticulated fine scale that gives the surface a white appearance *(A).* A close-up view demonstrates the fine white lacy scales known as Wickham's striae *(B).*

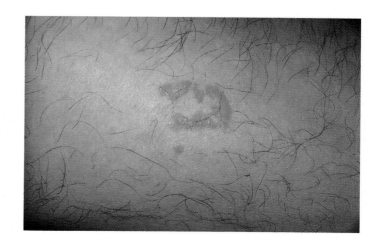

3.63
Lymphoma cutis.

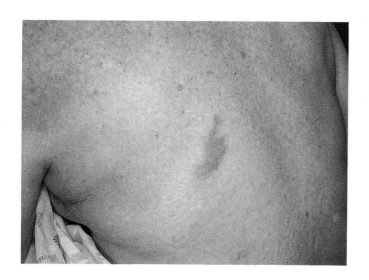

3.64
Metastatic breast carcinoma.

3.65
Alopecia mucinosa (follicular mucinosis). This erythematous to violaceous plaque resulted from infiltration of mucin into the follicular apparatus. Occasionally, this process is associated with or precedes the development of mycosis fungoides.

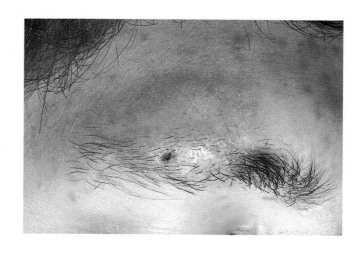

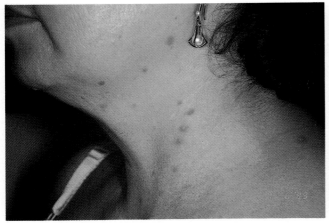

3.66
Lymphomatoid papulosis. This probably represents a clonal proliferation of T cells and may result in mycosis fungoides or another lymphoma.

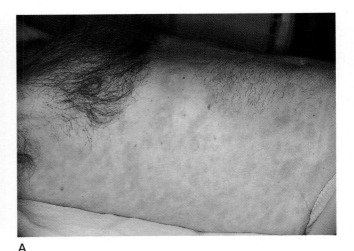

A

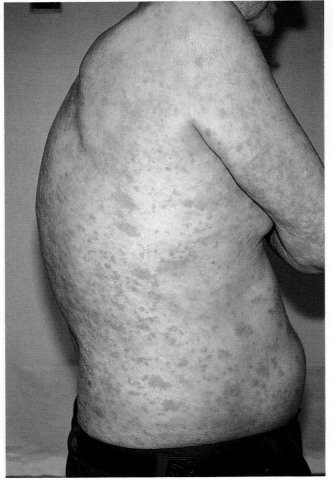

B

3.68
A, B, Mycosis fungoides or cutaneous T-cell lymphoma.

3.67
Small plaque parapsoriasis may be a pre—mycosis fungoides variant. These patients may be treated as though they had eczema or unusual psoriasis.

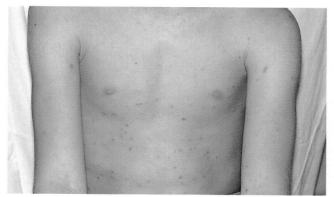

A

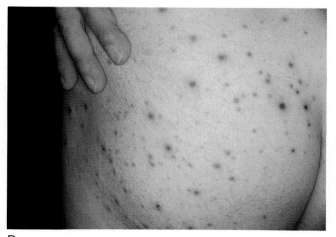

B

3.69

A, B, Pityriasis lichenoides et varioliformis acuta (PLEVA) or Mucha-Habermann disease. This disorder is characterized by small erythematous papules with central necrosis. Histopathologically it is a lymphocytic vasculitis. PLEVA is most often confused with insect bites.

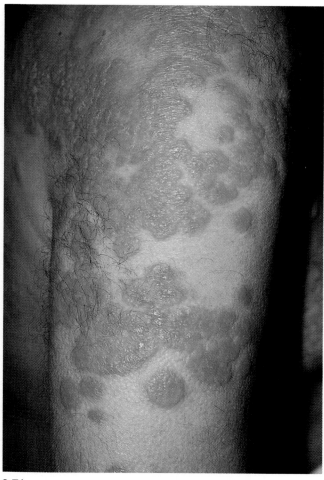

3.71

Sweet's syndrome (acute febrile neutrophilic dermatosis). This clinical lesion represents a massive infiltration of neutrophils within the dermis. Vascular destruction is not a feature. Some patients have associated leukemia.

3.70

Granuloma faciale. This erythematous facial plaque is a localized leukocytoclastic vasculitis.

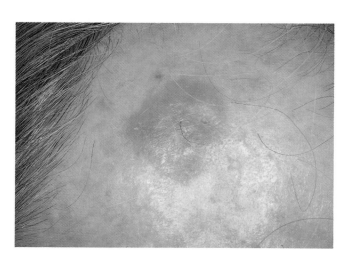

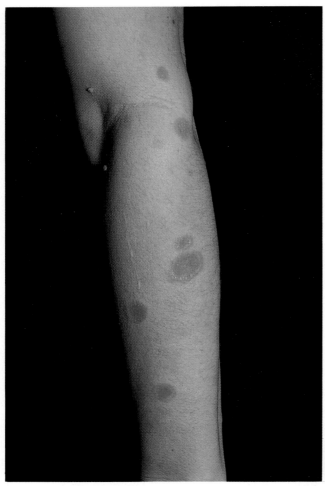

3.72
Sarcoidosis. Erythematous annular plaques.

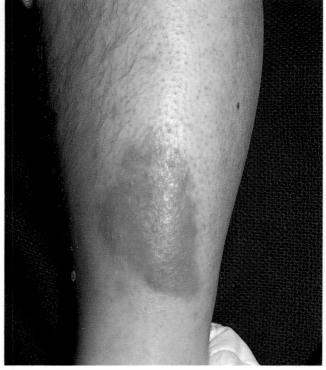

3.73
Pretibial myxedema. An erythematous plaque in a patient
with Graves' disease. This process is a manifestation of
mucin deposition in the dermis.

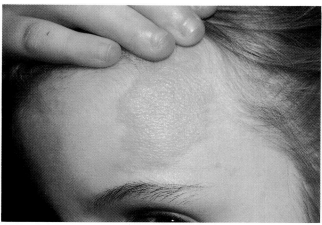

3.74
Tuberous sclerosis. Fibromatous plaque on the forehead.

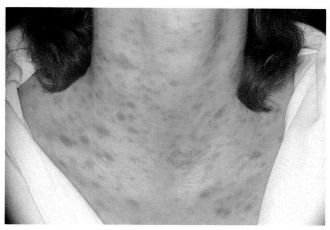

3.76
Urticaria pigmentosa. Erythematous fixed plaques that urticate with stroking (Darier's sign).

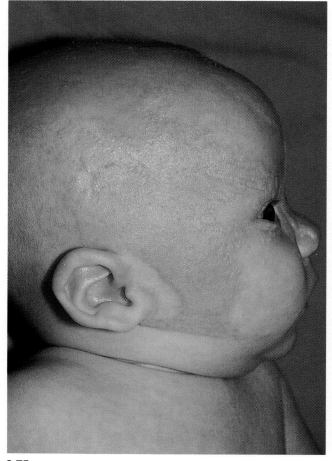

3.75
Nevus sebaceus of Jadassohn. A congenital lesion that becomes verrucous at puberty. Up to 15% of these patients develop basal cell carcinoma within the lesion. This patient has the epidermal nevus syndrome.

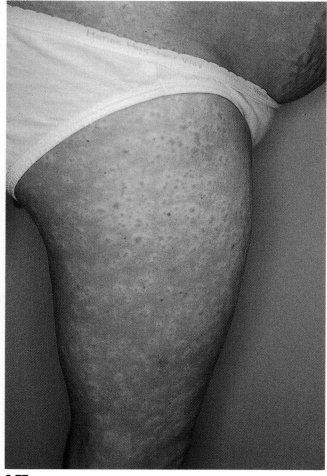

3.77
Pruritic urticarial papules and plaques of pregnancy (PUPPP). Multiple urticarial erythematous papules are seen in this near-term woman.

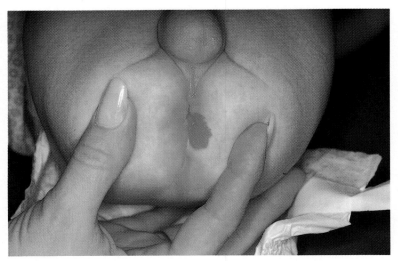

3.78
Capillary hemangioma.

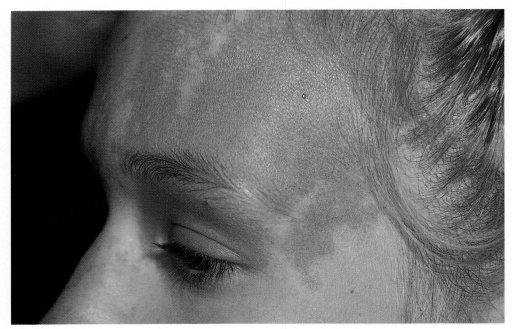

3.79
Port-wine stain. Dusky erythematous plaques.

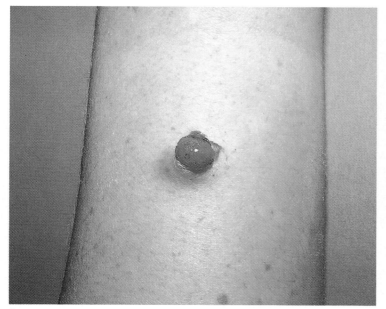

A

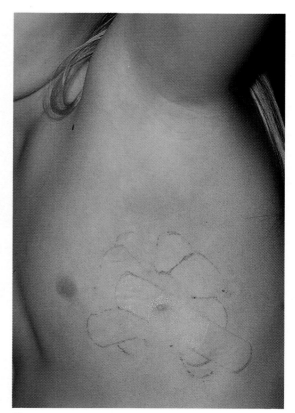

B

3.80

A, Pyogenic granuloma. A small papular lesion, which may develop after injury to the skin. *B,* Pyogenic granuloma with the "Band-Aid" sign. Because these lesions bleed with minor trauma, patients or their parents are inclined to layer on multiple Band-Aids.[5]

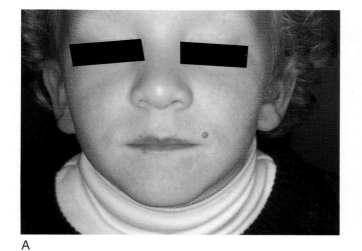

A

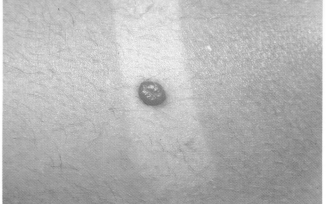

B

3.81

A, B, Spitz nevus (formerly known as benign juvenile melanoma) and also known as epithelioid cell–spindle cell nevomelanocytic nevus. This is a histologically bizarre but clinically benign lesion.

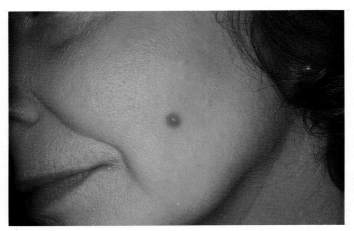

3.82
Metastatic malignant melanoma.

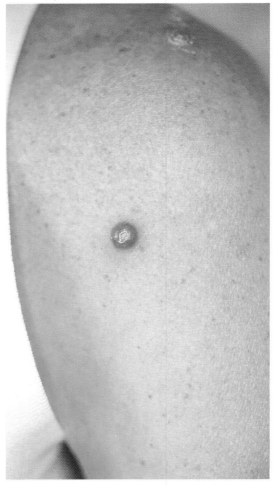

3.83
Bacillary angiomatosis in an HIV-positive patient.

BROWN OR TAN PAPULES AND PLAQUES

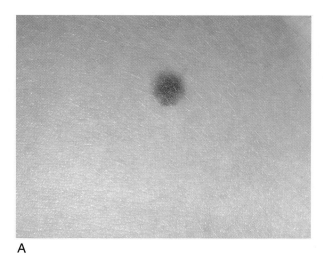

A

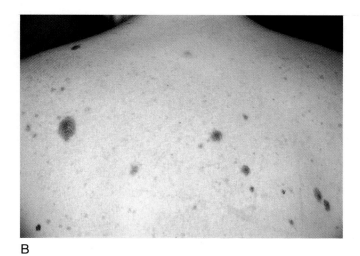

B

3.84
A, Compound melanocytic nevus. *B*, Multiple melanocytic nevi.

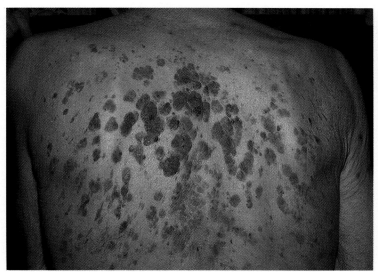

A

3.85
A, Multiple seborrheic keratoses. *B*, Irritated seborrheic keratoses
may become lighter in color.

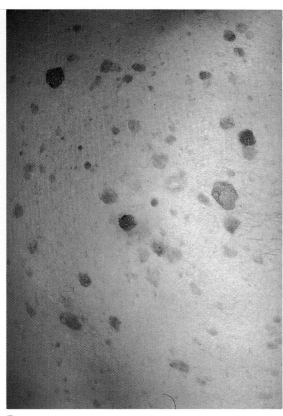

B

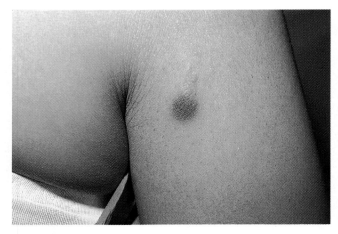

3.86
Dermatofibroma.

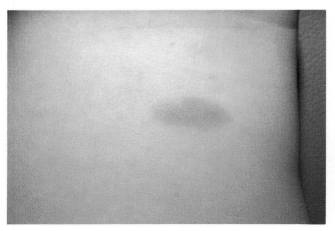

3.87
Urticaria pigmentosa. Solitary mastocytoma.

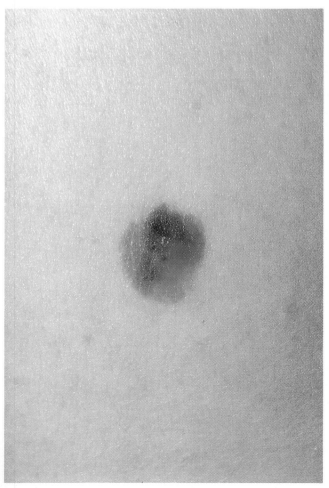

3.88
Malignant melanoma. Irregularly colored plaque.

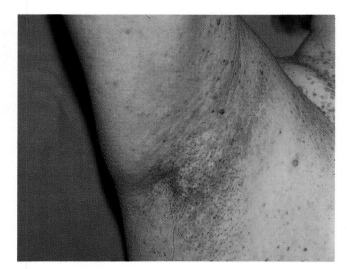

3.89
Acanthosis nigricans with multiple acrochordons and seborrheic keratoses. This patient had a gastric carcinoma.[5]

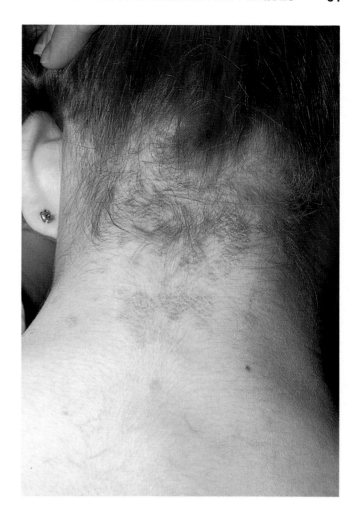

3.90
Confluent and reticulate papillomatosis. This simulates acanthosis nigricans but is unassociated with internal disease and is reticulated.

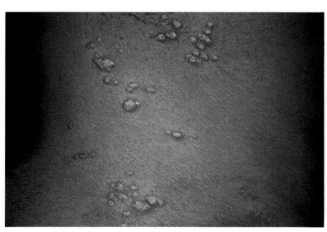

3.91
Sarcoidosis. Tan, hyperpigmented papules and plaques.

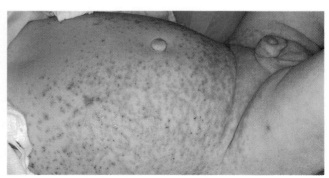

3.92
Letterer-Siwe variant of histiocytosis X. Hemorrhagic, tan papular lesions.

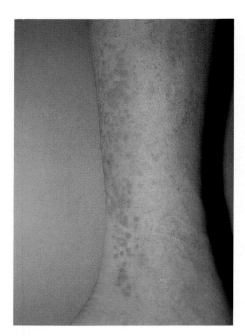

3.93
Lichen amyloidosus.

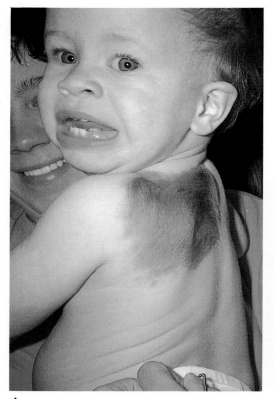

A

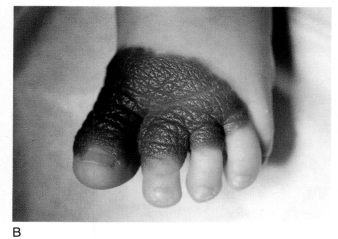

B

3.94
A, B, Congenital melanocytic nevus.

BLUE-BLACK PAPULES AND PLAQUES

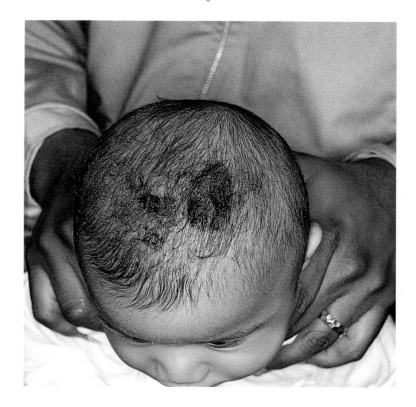

3.95
Congenital melanocytic nevus.

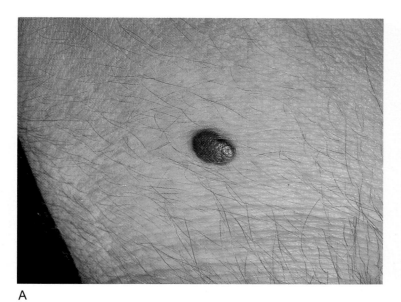

A

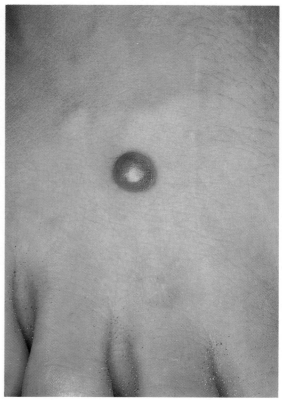

B

3.96
A, B, Blue nevus. A uniform, dark blue papule.[2]

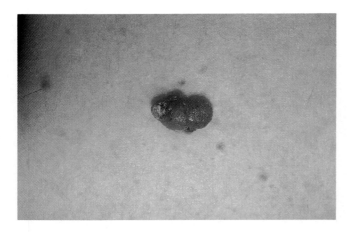

3.97
Malignant melanoma.

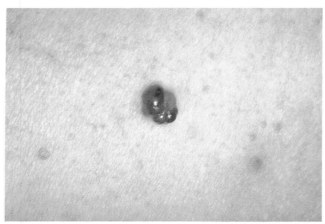

3.98
Pigmented basal cell carcinoma. A rare manifestation of basal cell carcinoma.

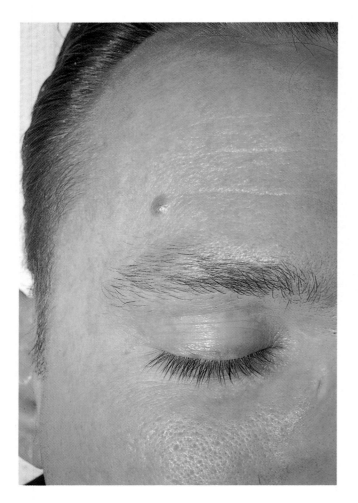

3.99
Eccrine spiradenoma. A rare, often painful adnexal tumor.

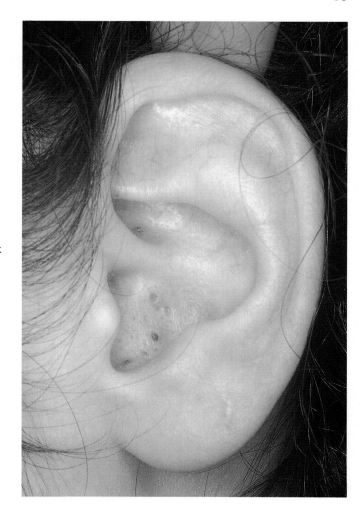

3.100
Comedones in acne vulgaris. These papules have a black expressible core (blackheads).

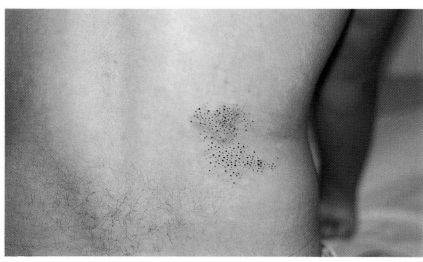

3.101
Nevus comedonicus. An epidermal nevoid lesion consisting of multiple open comedones.

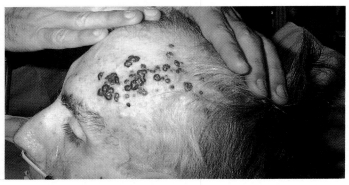

3.102
Metastatic malignant melanoma.

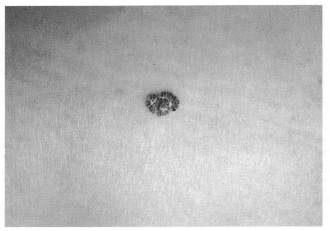

A

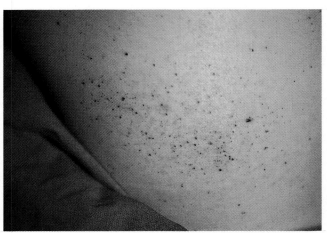

B

3.103
A, Angiokeratomas. A, Solitary lesion. B, Multiple pin-point pigmented papules in Fabry's disease (angiokera-toma corporis diffusum). C, Multiple lesions known as angiokeratomas of Mibelli.

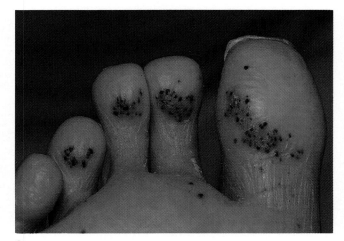

C

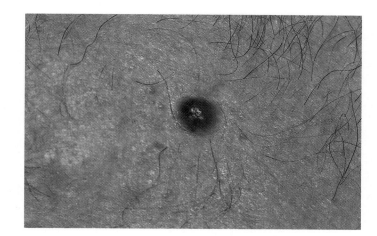

3.104
Capillary hemangioma.[5]

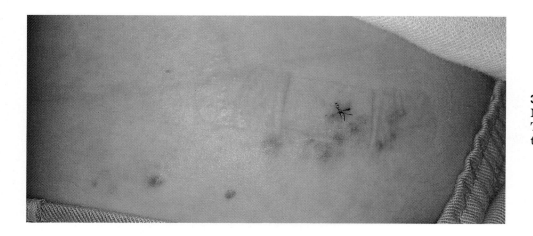

3.105
Multiple glomus tumors. These are vascular tumors that may at times be painful.

3.106
Capillary-lymphatic malformations (hemolymphangiomas) in a patient with Klippel-Trenaunay-Weber syndrome.

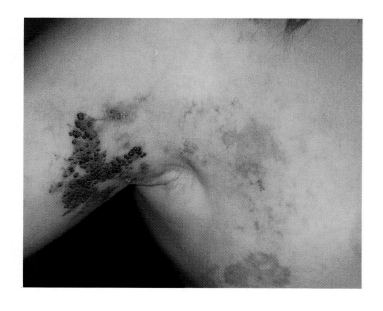

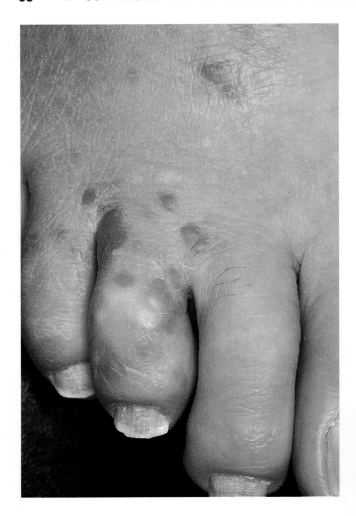

3.107
Classic Kaposi's sarcoma, non-HIV, in an elderly male.

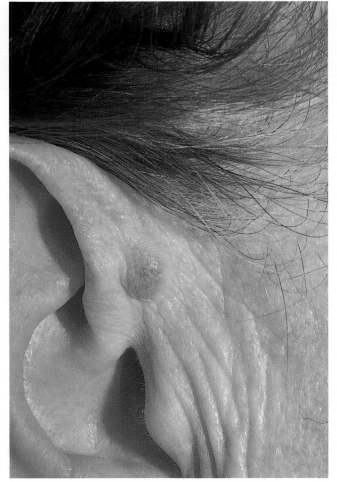

3.108
Venous lake.

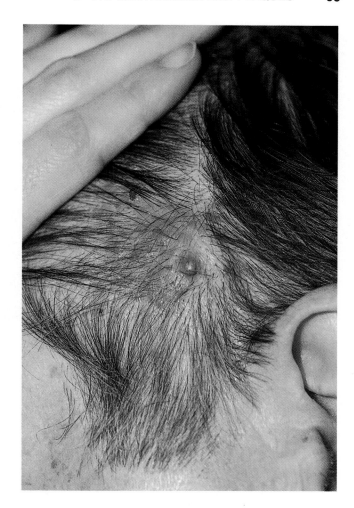

3.109
Angiolymphoid hyperplasia with eosinophilia or pseudo-pyogenic granuloma (Kimura's disease).

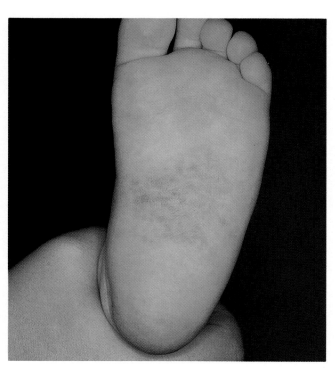

3.110
Venous varicosities in a patient with Klippel-Trenaunay-Weber syndrome.

YELLOW PAPULES AND PLAQUES

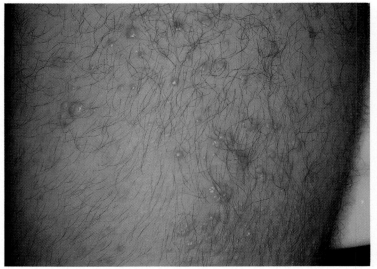

A

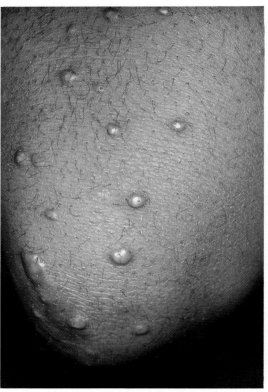

B

3.111
A, B, Eruptive xanthomas.

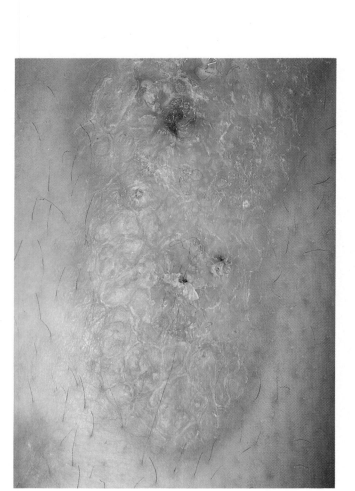

3.112
Necrobiosis lipoidica diabeticorum. Erythematous to yellow plaque, most often on the anterior leg. Most of these patients have diabetes mellitus.

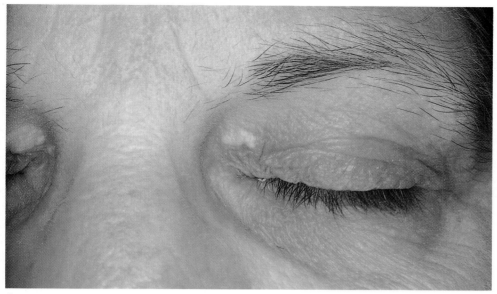

A

3.113
A, B, Xanthelasma. Planar xanthomas on the eyelid. The patient in *B* was normolipemic.

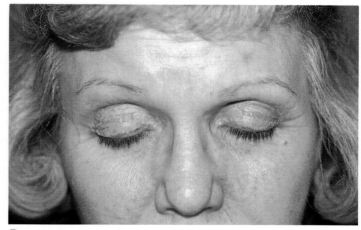

B

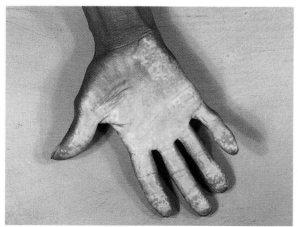

A

B

3.114
A, Plane xanthoma on the palmar surface. *B,* Generalized plane xanthoma in a patient with paraproteinemia.

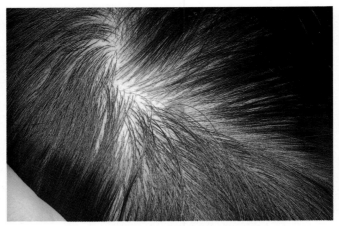

3.115
Juvenile xanthogranuloma. This lesion resolves spontaneously during childhood.

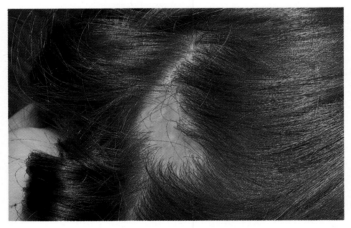

3.116
Nevus sebaceus of Jadassohn.

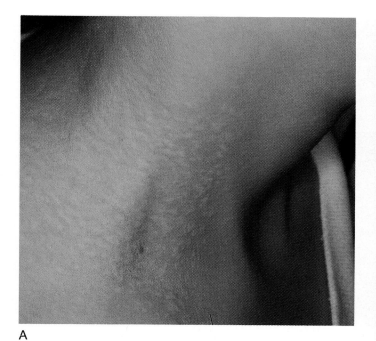

A

3.117
A, B, Pseudoxanthoma elasticum. This disease has a variety
of inheritance patterns. Yellowish papules are observed in
flexural skin. Patients develop premature vascular disease.

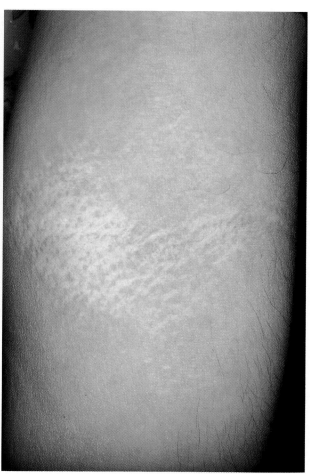

B

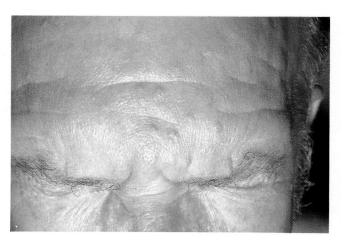

3.118
Sebaceous nevi (senile sebaceous hyperplasia).

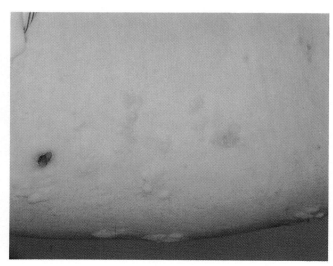

3.119
Nevus lipomatosus.

PAPULES OR PLAQUES WITH PROMINENT SURFACE CHANGES

In Characteristic Locations

Breast

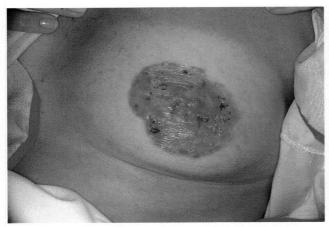

3.120
Paget's disease of the breast. This is associated with ductal adenocarcinoma of the breast.

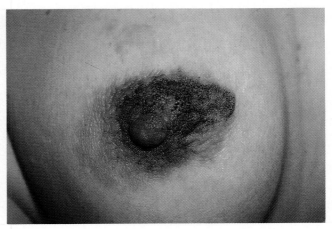

3.121
Hyperkeratosis of the nipple. This is a benign verrucous change.

Sun-Exposed

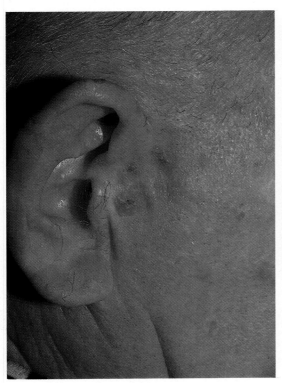

A

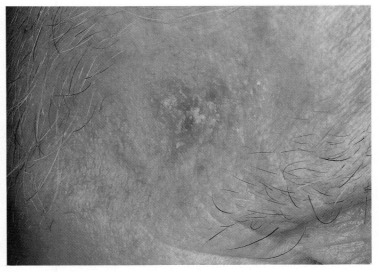

B

3.122
A, Multiple actinic keratoses. *B*, Actinic keratosis.

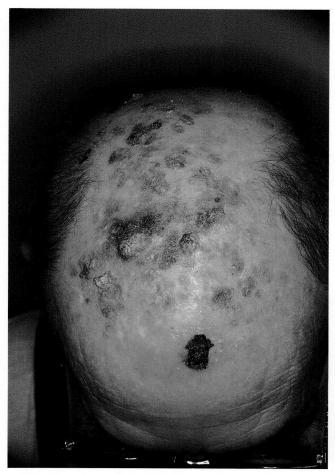

3.123
Multiple squamous cell carcinomas.[5]

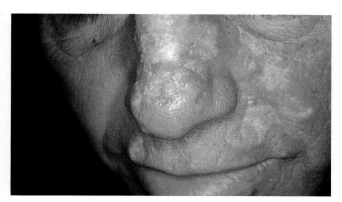

3.124
Hypertrophic discoid lupus erythematosus with prominent adherent scale.

Scattered

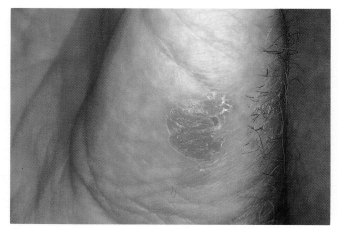

A

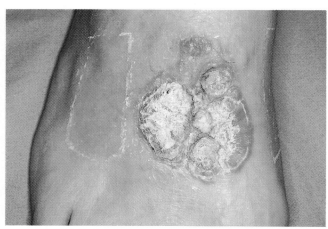

B

3.125
A, B, Bowen's disease. In situ squamous cell carcinoma. *A,*[8]. *B,*[2].

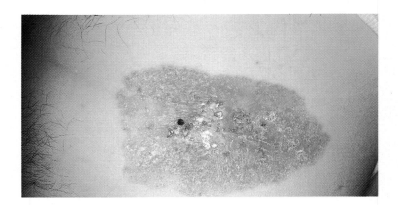

3.126
Superficial basal cell epithelioma.

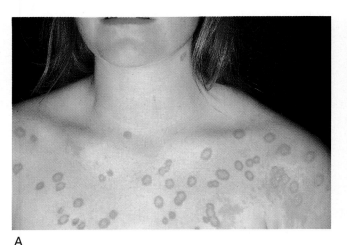

A

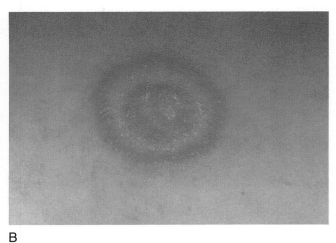

B

3.127
A, B, Tinea corporis. Annular scaly plaques in superficial basal cell epithelioma.

3.128
Tinea capitis.

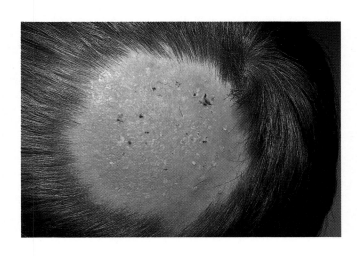

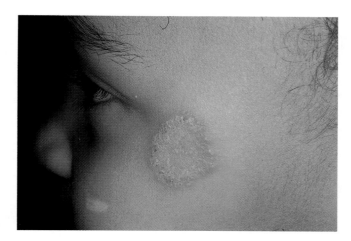

3.129
Tinea faciale.

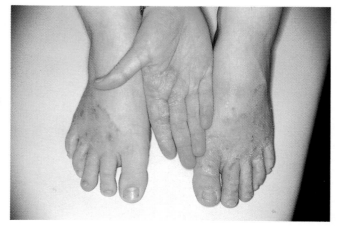

3.130
Chronic *Trichophyton rubrum* infection. Two-foot, one-hand disease.

3.131
Inflammatory linear verrucous epidermal nevus.[3]

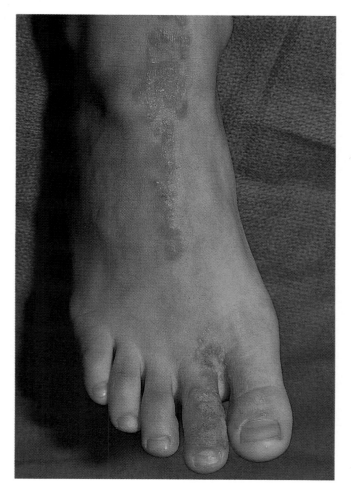

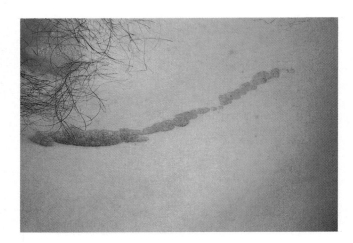

3.132
Linear epidermal nevus.

3.133
Ichthyosis hystrix. An epidermal nevus variant.

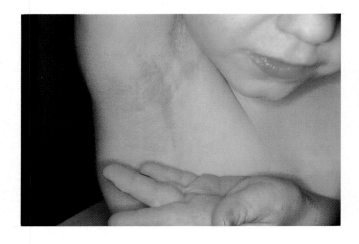

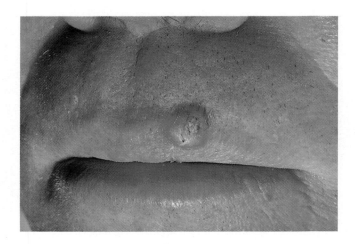

3.134
Keratoacanthoma. This lesion occurs suddenly, developing within weeks to months. It is a benign, epithelial neoplasm, but its fast growth characteristic can be quite destructive.

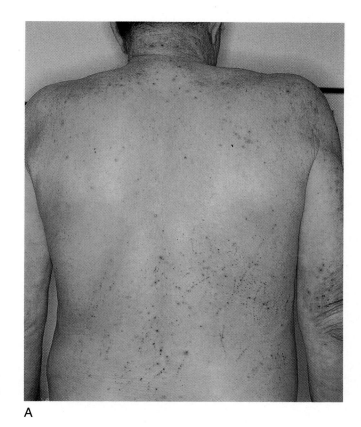

3.135

A, Neurodermatitis. Multiple excoriated, slightly scaly papules. Note the sparing on the area of the back where the patient is unable to reach. *B,* Neurodermatitis.

A

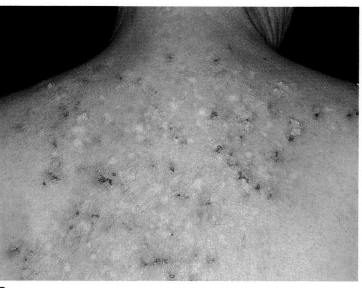

B

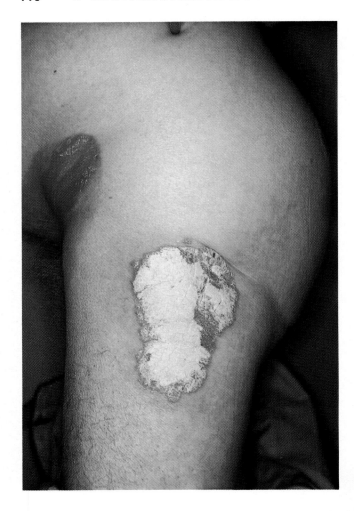

3.136
Psoriasis vulgaris. Thick micaceous scale on an erythematous plaque.

3.137
Seborrheic dermatitis.

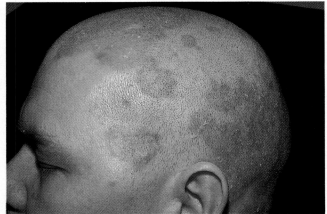

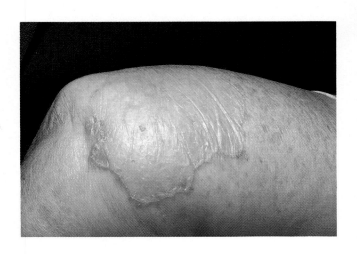

3.138
Porokeratosis. An unusual lesion in which there is a scaly wall near the periphery (this is known as a cornoid lamella). Carcinoma occasionally develops in porokeratotic lesions.

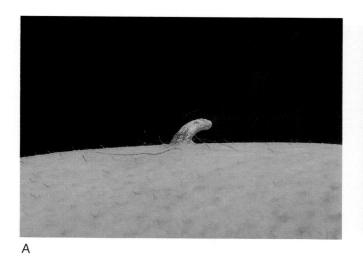

A

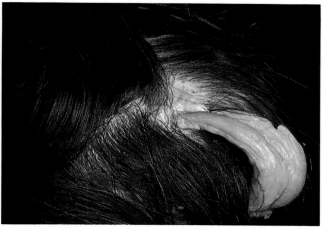

B

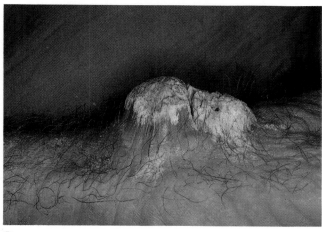

C

3.139
Cutaneous horn. *A,* In this case the horn represented a viral wart. *B,* This example is due to an actinic keratosis. *C,* This case is due to a squamous cell carcinoma. *C,*[2].

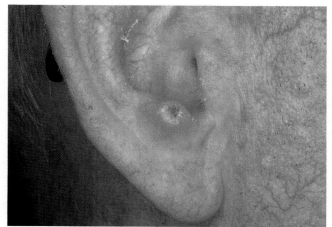

A

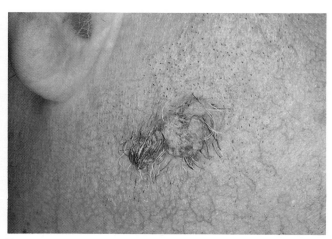

B

3.140
A, B, Squamous cell carcinoma of the skin.

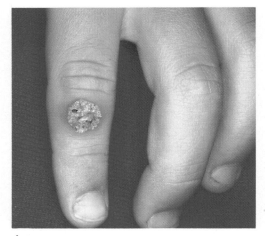

A

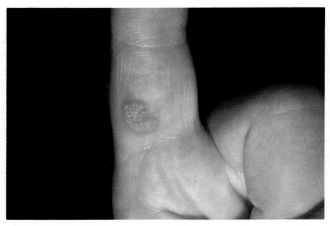

B

3.141
A, B, Verruca vulgaris.

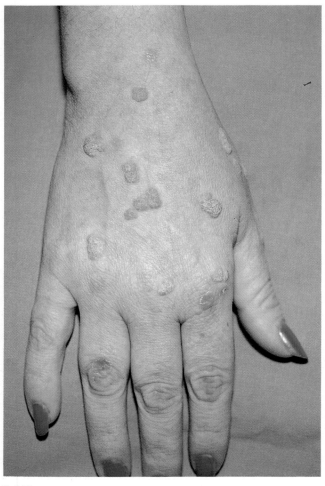

3.142
Multiple warts in an immunosuppressed transplant patient.[2]

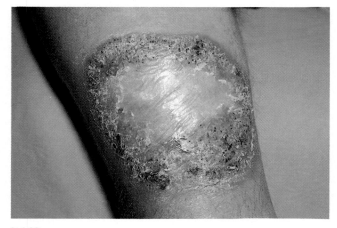

3.143
Blastomycosis. This verrucous plaque is a manifestation of a deep fungal infection.

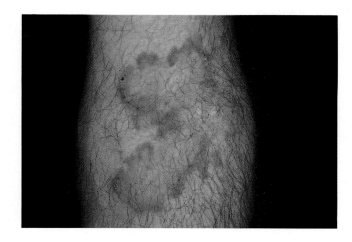

3.144
Elastosis perforans serpiginosa. This scaly serpentine plaque is caused by perforation of elastic tissue through the epidermis.

3.145
Perforating folliculitis.

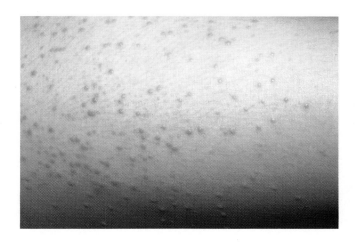

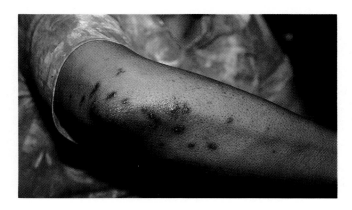

3.146
Kyrle's disease in a diabetic patient on hemodialysis. This is another perforating dermatosis.

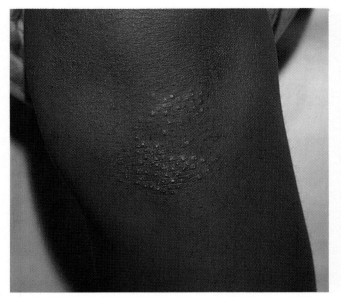

3.147
Lichen spinulosus.[3]

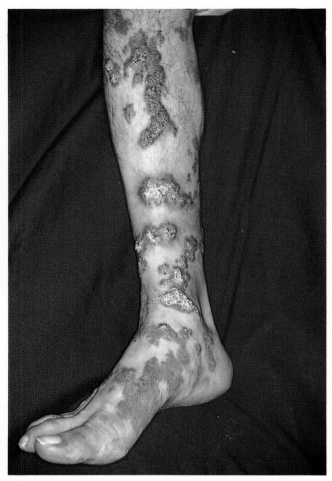

3.149
Angiokeratomas with prominent surface change.[6]

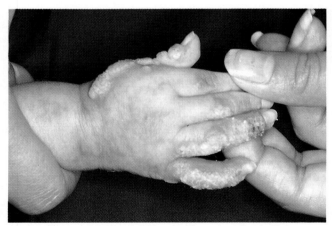

3.148
Incontinentia pigmenti: verrucous stage.[6]

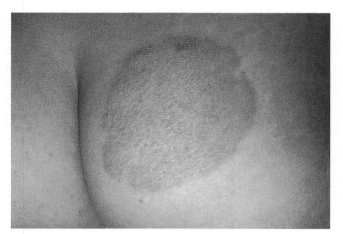

3.150
Parapsoriasis en plaques.

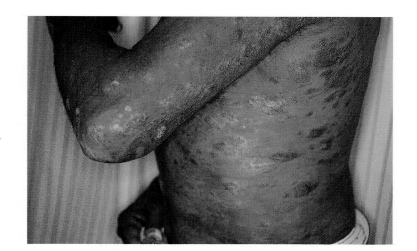

3.151
Mycosis fungoides (cutaneous T-cell lymphoma).

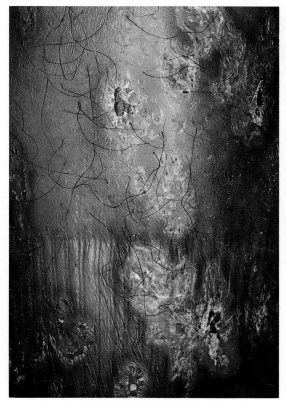

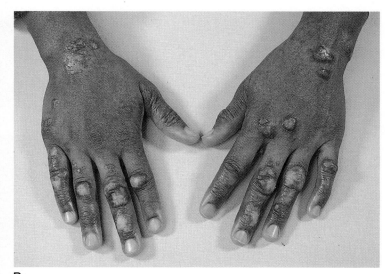

B

A

3.152
A, B, Sarcoidosis.

OFTEN SYMMETRIC

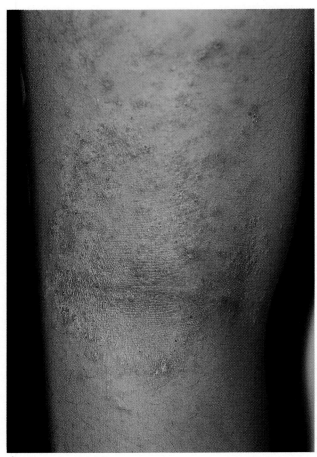

A

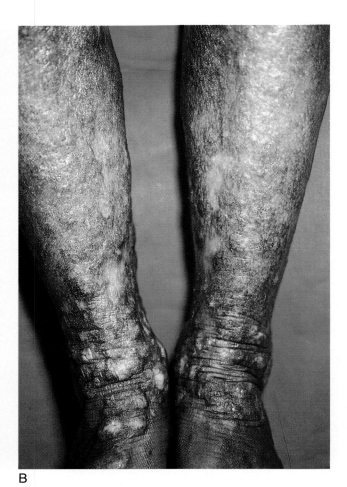

B

3.153
A to *C*, Atopic dermatitis.

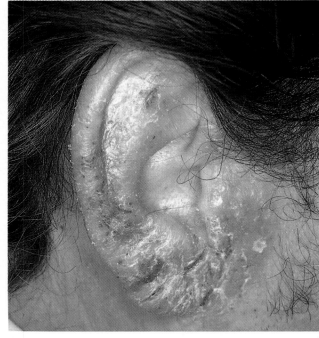

C

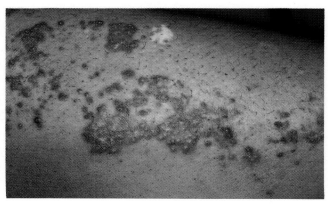

3.154
Darier's disease (keratosis follicularis). An autosomal dominant disorder. The lesions are keratotic papules. Sunlight seems to exacerbate this disease, as seen in this patient.

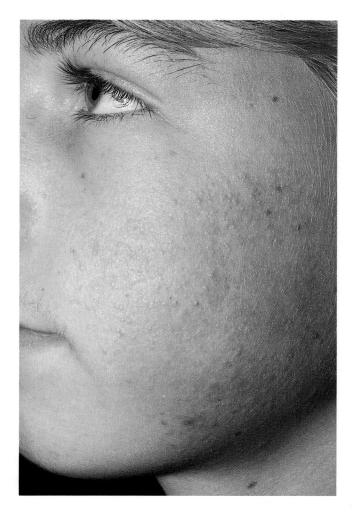

3.155
Keratosis pilaris. Perifollicular hyperkeratotic papules. This common disorder is probably associated with atopy, and may respond to keratolytic agents.

3.156
Hypertrophic lichen planus.

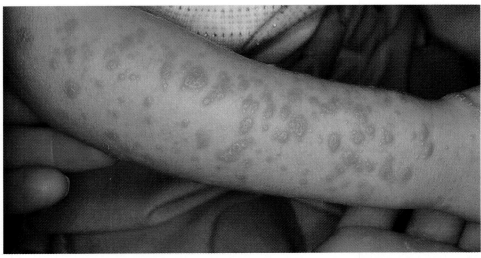

A

3.157
A, B, Lichen planus. The fine reticulated white scales (Wickham's striae) are prominently displayed.

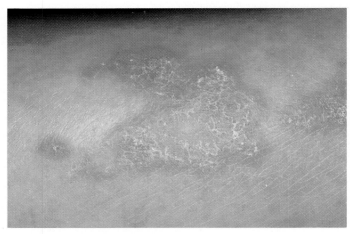

B

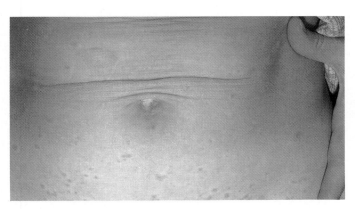

3.158
Pityriasis rosea. Fine scale is seen just inside the border.

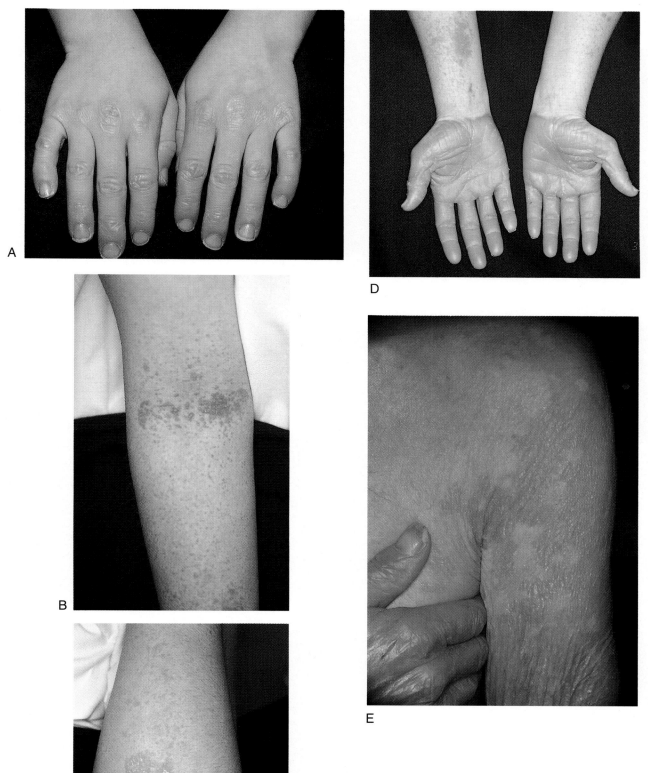

3.159

A to *E*, Pityriasis rubra pilaris. An idiopathic psoriasis-like condition characterized by scaly plaques (*A* and *B*), perifollicular lesions *(C)*, palmoplantar hyperkeratosis *(D)*, and islands of "normal" skin within the generalized erythroderma *(E)*.

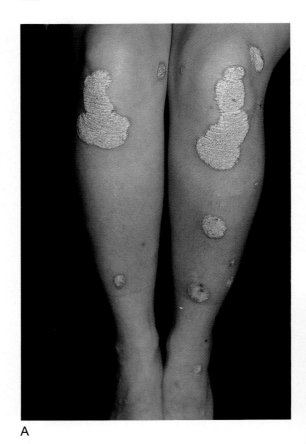

A

3.160
A to *C*, Psoriasis vulgaris.

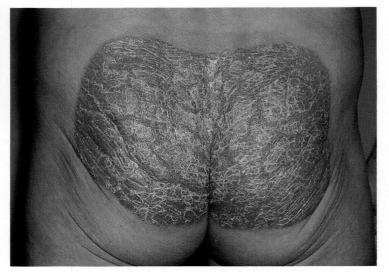

B

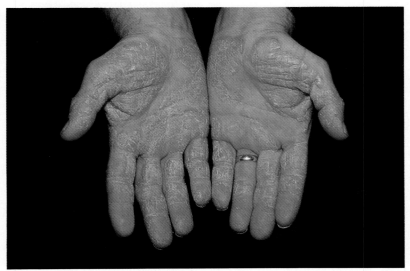

C

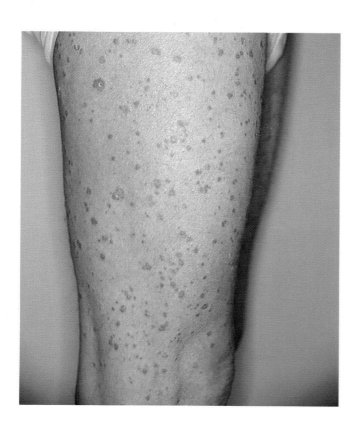

3.161
Guttate psoriasis.[2]

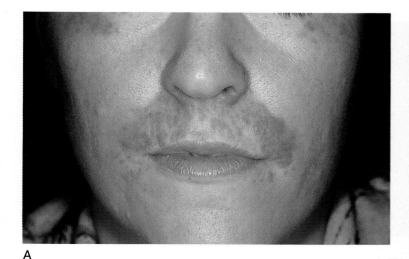

A

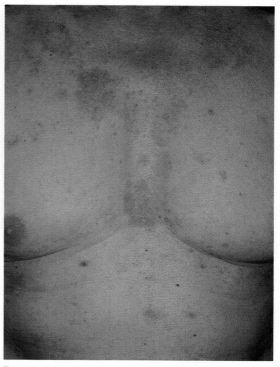

B

3.162
A, B, Seborrheic dermatitis. Erythema with "greasy"-looking scale in a seborrheic distribution (scalp, eyebrows, nasolabial fold, perioral area, midchest, and groin).

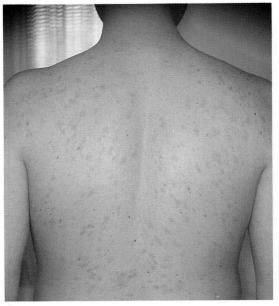

A

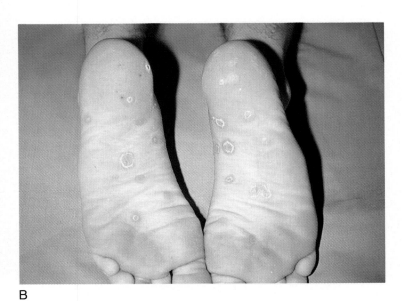

B

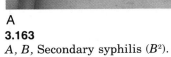

A, B, Secondary syphilis (*B*²).

3.164
Tinea versicolor.

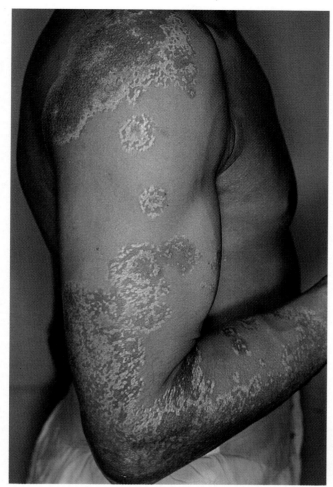

3.165
Lichen sclerosus et atrophicus.

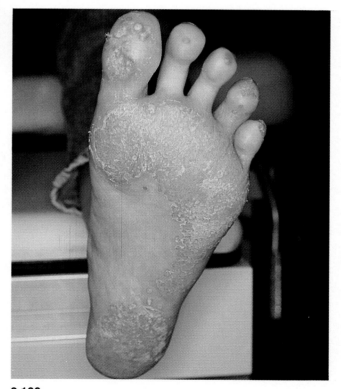

3.166
Reiter's disease. This psoriasis-like dermatitis is triggered by nongonococcal urethritis or enteritis. It is associated with uveitis and spondylitis or sacroiliitis. Patients are usually male, and there is a high prevalence of HLA-B27.

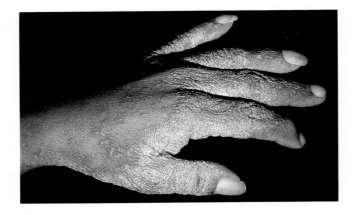

3.167
Norwegian variant of scabies. These patients are often immunosuppressed or have psychiatric problems. They develop a hyperkeratotic variant that contains multiple mites and is highly transmissible.[11]

3.168
Chondrodermatitis nodularis helicis. A process in which the cartilage degenerates.

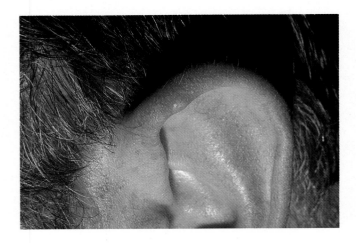

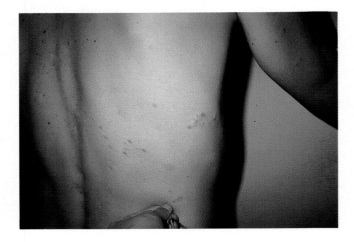

3.169
Leiomyomas. Multiple erythematous, painful dermal tumors.

NODULES AND TUMORS OF THE SKIN

These are infiltrative processes which are either inflammatory, infectious or neoplastic. They are best separated by their color.

FLESH-COLORED NODULES AND TUMORS

Cystic Lesions

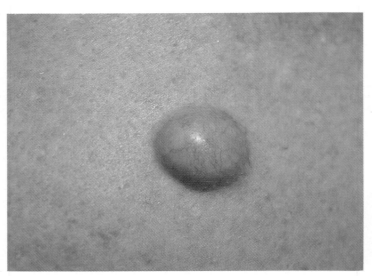

A

4.1

A, B, Epidermal cyst. C, Epidermal cyst in a patient with Gardner's syndrome. This combines epidermal cysts with familial polyposis coli. It is inherited as an autosomal dominant trait. The polyps are adenomatous and there is a high incidence of colon cancer.

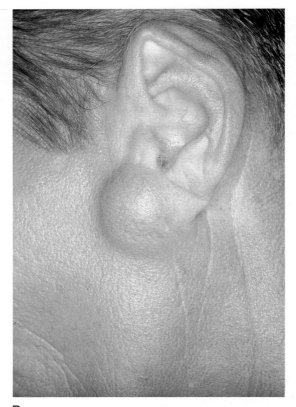

B

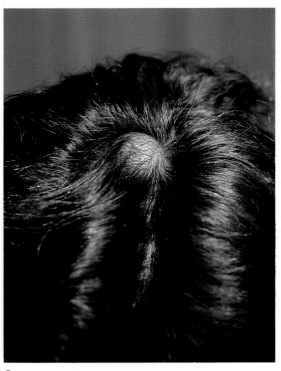

C

4.2
Pilar cyst.

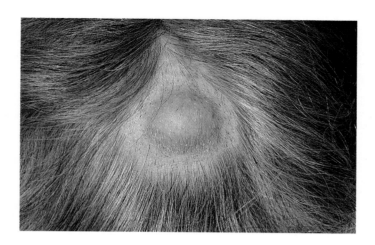

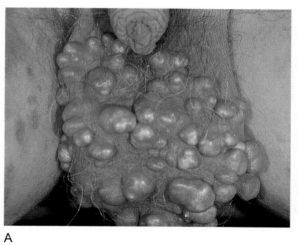

A

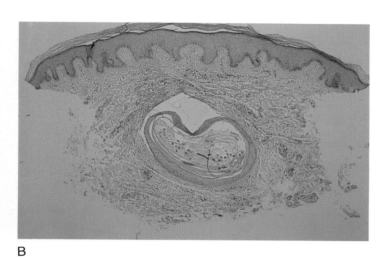

B

4.3
A, Multiple scrotal cysts. *B*, Histopathology of a small cyst reveals an epithelial lining filled with semisolid keratinous debris.

4.4
Ganglion cyst.

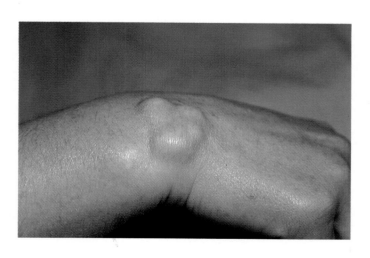

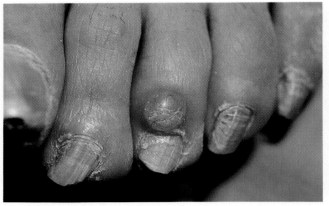

4.5
Myxoid cyst or mucinous pseudocyst. This lesion does not have an epithelial lining. It may communicate with the joint space, and if opened it exudes a mucin-like material.

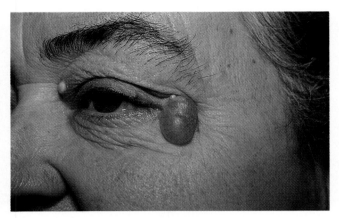

4.6
Hidrocystoma.

Solid Tumors

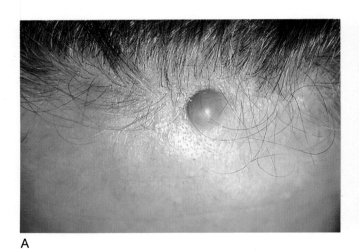

A

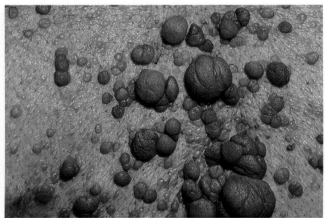

B

4.7
A, Solitary neurofibroma. *B*, Neurofibromas in neurofibromatosis.

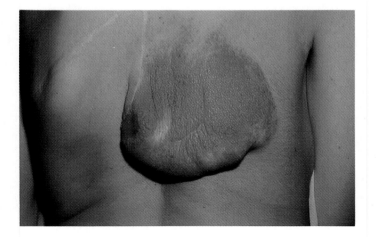

4.8
Large neurofibroma.

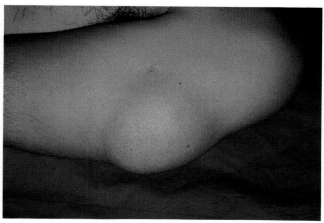

4.9
Lipoma.

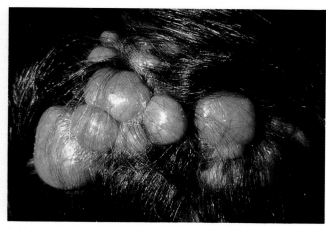

4.10
Cylindromas or turban tumors.

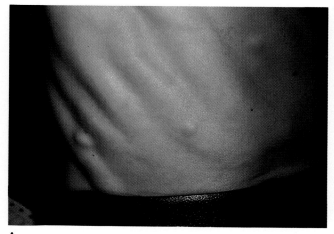

A

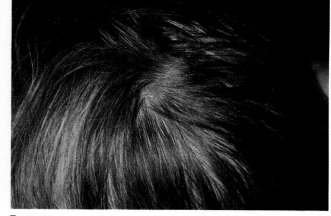

B

4.11
A, Metastatic carcinoma from a laryngeal squamous cell carcinoma. *B,* Metastatic breast carcinoma. *C,* Histopathologic appearance of metastatic breast cancer.

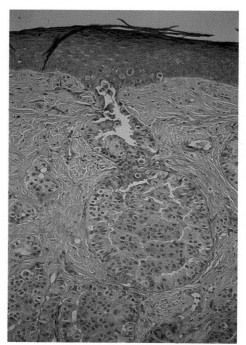

C

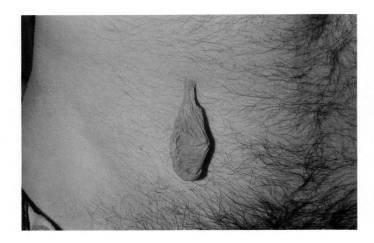

4.12
Large skin tag (acrochordon).

4.13
Deep or subcutaneous granuloma annulare.

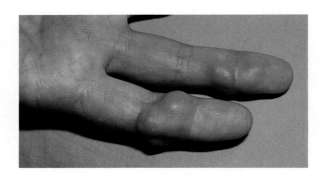

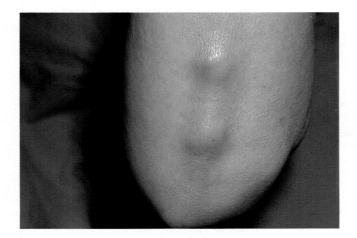

4.14
Rheumatoid nodules. Subcutaneous nodules on the extensor surface of the arm near the elbow, in a patient with rheumatoid arthritis.

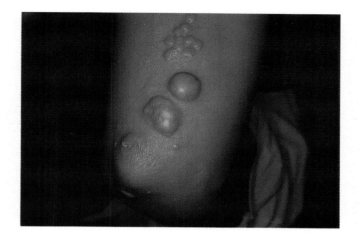

4.15
Tuberous xanthomas. These were associated with an elevated cholesterol level in Type II hyperlipoprotein-emia.

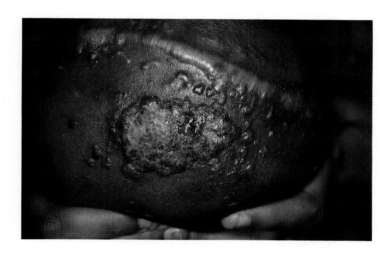

4.16
A, Multiple lymphangioma circumscriptum (lymphatic malformation) on a partially amputated extremity. *B*, Histopathologic appearance of this condition demonstrates the dilated lymphatics.

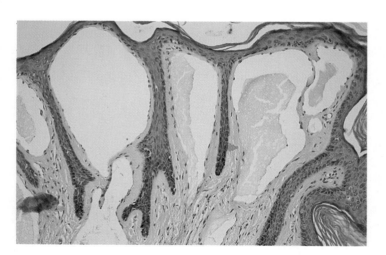

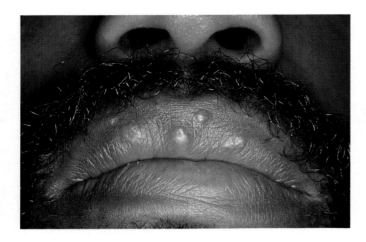

4.17
Sarcoidosis.

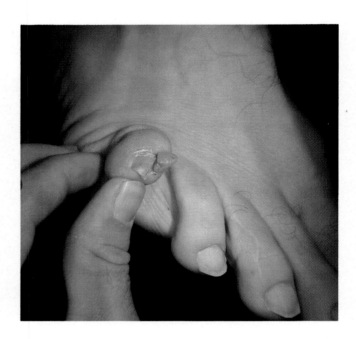

4.18
A, Acquired digital fibrous tumor. A nodular infiltrate of fibrous tissue that may resolve spontaneously.[10] *B,* Acquired digital fibroma.

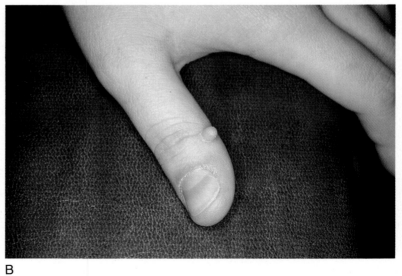

B

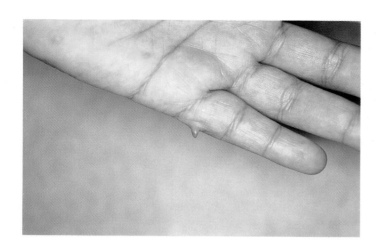

4.19
Rudimentary digit.

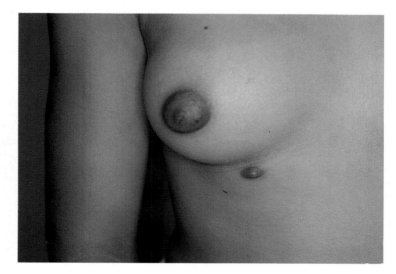

4.20
Accessory nipple.

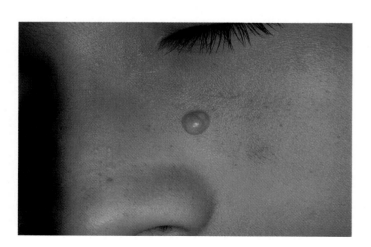

4.21
Pilomatricoma.[2]

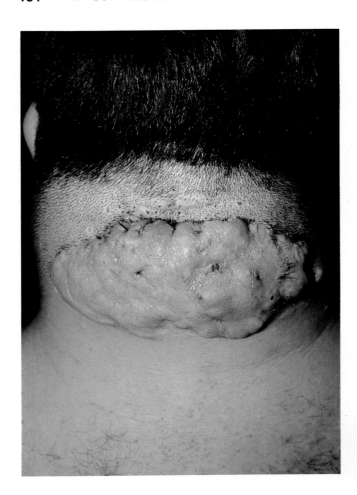

4.22
Acne keloidalis nuchae. These perifollicular inflammatory lesions result in keloid formation. They tend to be limited to the nuchal area and are most often observed in black men.

4.23
Keloid after ear piercing.

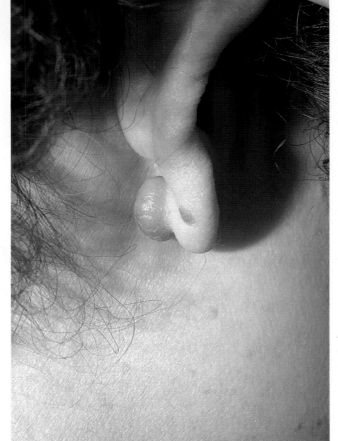

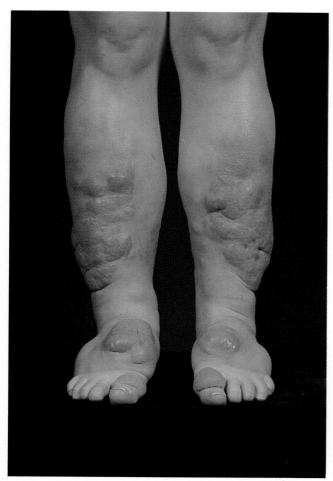

4.24
Pretibial myxedema.

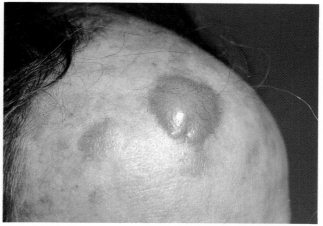

A

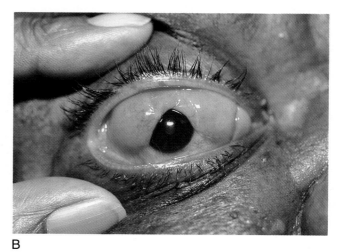

B

4.25
A, B, Lymphoma cutis.

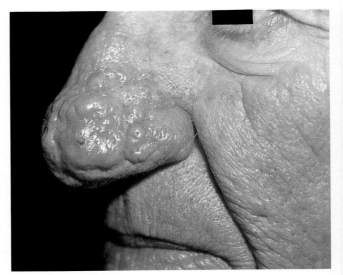

A

4.26
A, Rhinophyma formation in a patient with acne rosacea.
B, Massive lesion of rhinophyma.

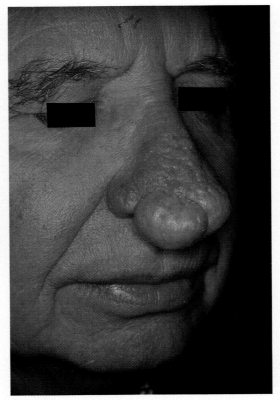

B

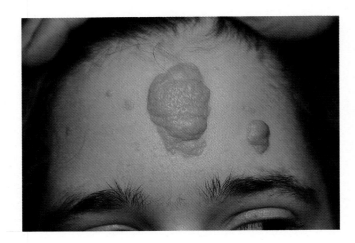

4.27
Angiofibroma in a patient with tuberous sclerosis.

4.28
Multiple calluses.

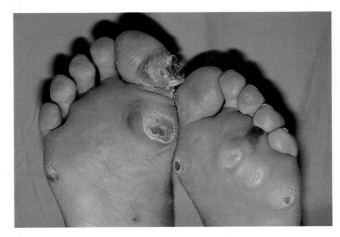

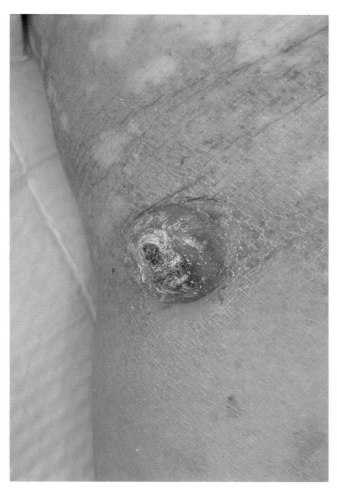

4.29
Amelanotic melanoma.[2]

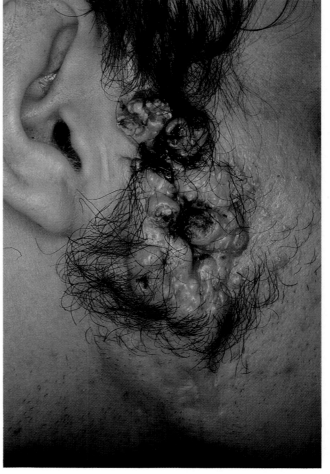

4.30
Nevus sebaceus. Large cystic and solid tumors are present.

ERYTHEMATOUS NODULES AND TUMORS

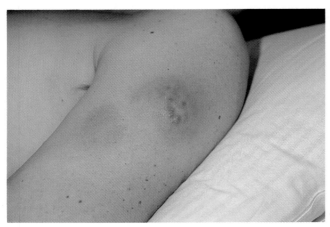

4.31
Panniculitis in a patient with alpha-1-antitrypsin deficiency. Panniculitis consists of inflammation in the subcutaneous tissue and results in a deep-seated nodule that is often tender.

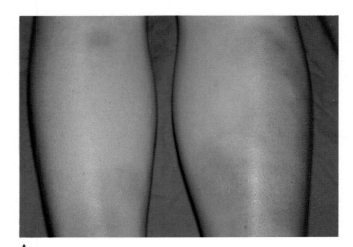

A

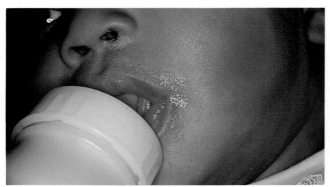

4.32
Panniculitis in a child induced by cold.

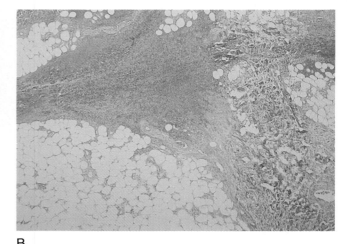

B

4.33
A, Erythema nodosum. The most common form of panniculitis. Most common etiologic or associated disorders include drugs (antibiotics or oral contraceptives), infections (streptococcal or deep fungal), sarcoidosis, and inflammatory bowel disease. *B,* Histopathologic appearance of erythema nodosum demonstrates the septal panniculitis.

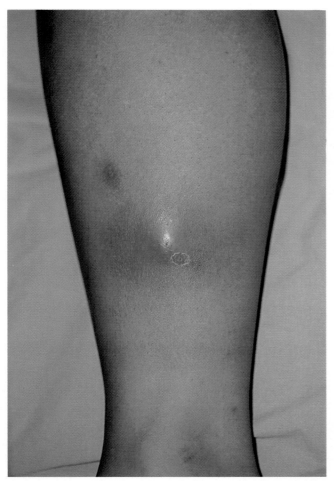

4.34
Furuncle due to *Staphylococcus aureus* infection.

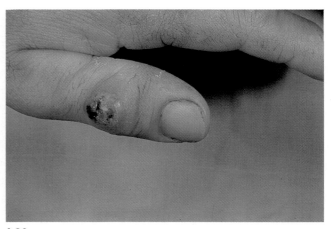

4.36
Milker's nodule.[5]

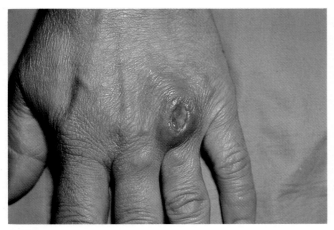

4.35
Atypical mycobacterial infection due to *Mycobacterium marinum* acquired from a fish tank. This primary inoculation site may be followed by a sporotrichoid (lymphangitic) spread of lesions up the arm.

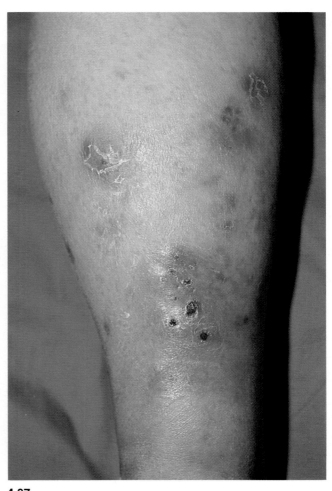

4.37
Erythema induratum is a manifestation of infection with *Mycobacterium tuberculosis*.

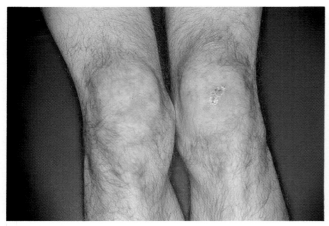

4.38
Nodular vasculitis. Deep-seated nodules in this patient, who also has a livedo reticularis pattern.

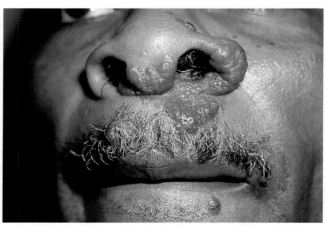

4.40
Sarcoidosis.

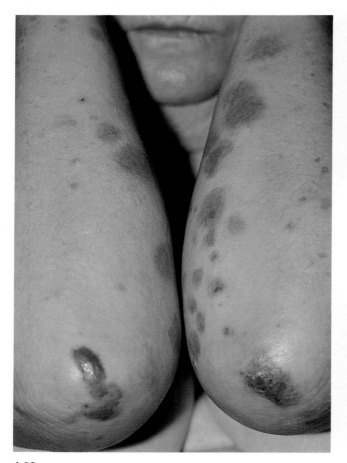

4.39
Erythema elevatum diutinum. A localized form of chronic leukocytoclastic vasculitis.[5]

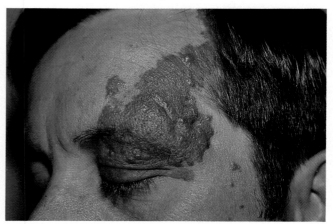

4.41
Superficial hemangioma.

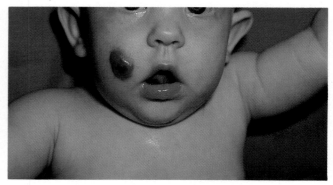

4.42
Superficial hemangioma.

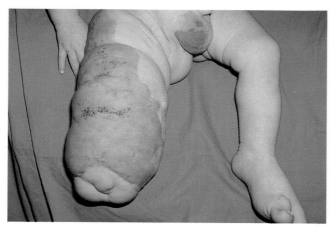

4.43
Lymphangioma with lymphedema.

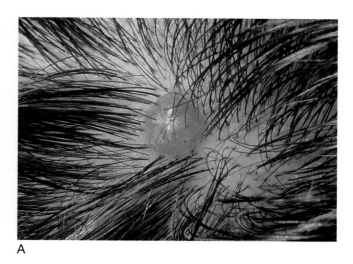

A

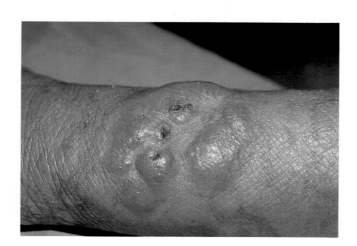

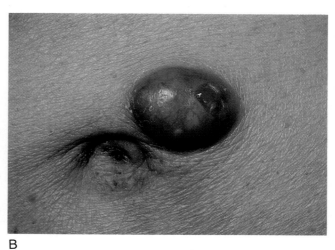

B
4.45
A, Metastatic malignant melanoma. *B*, Metastatic gastric carcinoma. This periumbilical location was noted by Sister Mary Joseph at the Mayo Clinic and has been termed a Sister Mary Joseph nodule.[11]

4.44
Clear cell acanthoma.

4.46
Mycosis fungoides. Tumor formation is usually a late event.

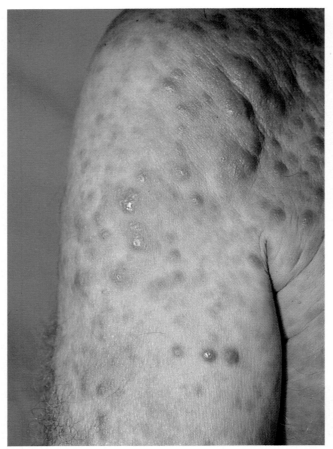

4.47
Patients with chronic myelocytic leukemia can form cutaneous nodules on rare occasions.

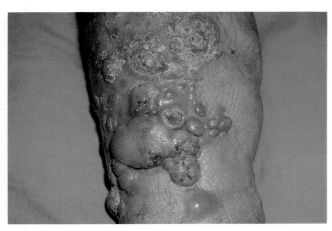

4.49
Squamous cell carcinoma arising in a burn scar: Marjolin's ulcer.

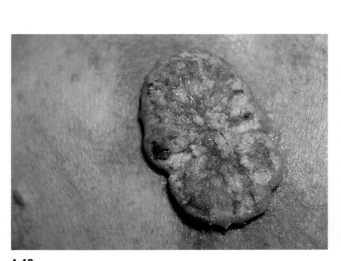

4.48
Squamous cell carcinoma.

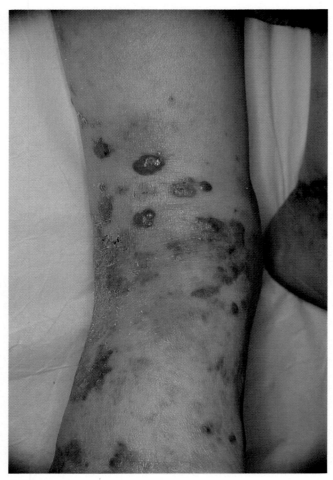

4.50
Tumors of classic Kaposi's sarcoma.

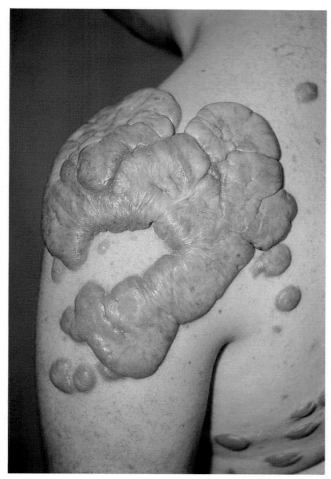

4.51
Keloid.

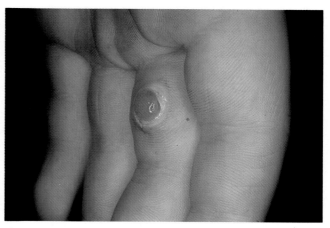

4.53
Pyogenic granuloma. The lesions often have a collar or moat.

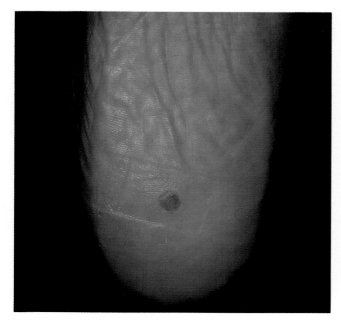

4.52
Eccrine poroma.

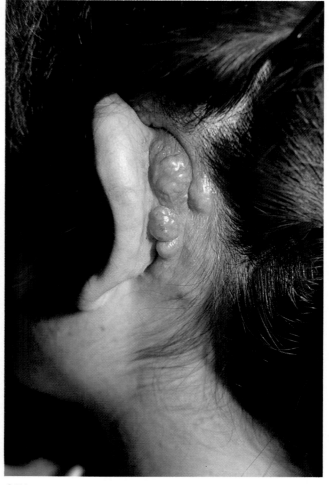

4.54
Angiolymphoid hyperplasia with eosinophilia or pseudo-pyogenic granuloma.

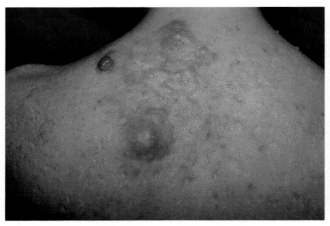

4.55
Dermatofibrosarcoma protuberans. This lesion frequently recurs locally but rarely metastasizes.

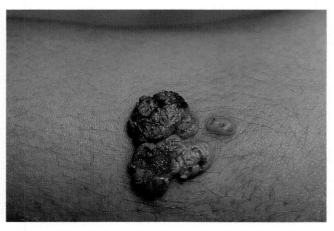

4.57
Syringocystadenoma papilliferum.

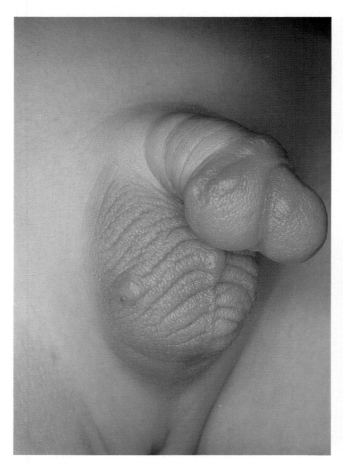

4.56
Nodular lesions of scabies.

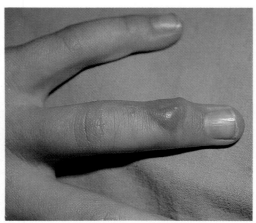

4.58
Juvenile fibromatosis.

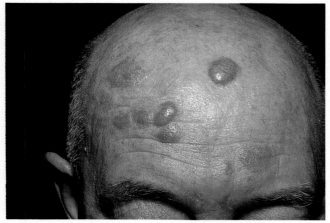

4.59
Benign lymphocytic infiltrate.

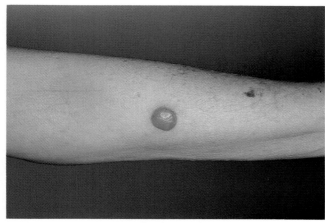

4.60
Non-Hodgkin's T-cell lymphoma.

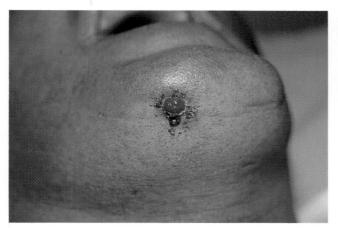

4.61
Dental sinus. This lesion forms a tract to a periapical abscess. *Actinomyces* species often grow.

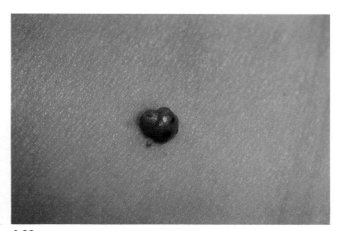

4.62
Clear cell hidradenoma.

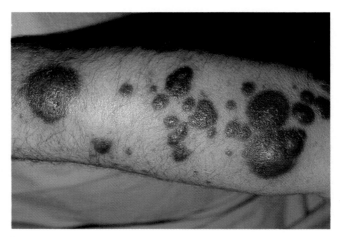

4.63
Acute febrile neutrophilic dermatosis (Sweet's syndrome). The purpuric nature of this patient's lesion relates to the associated thrombocytopenia.

BROWN, BLUE, OR BLACK NODULES AND TUMORS

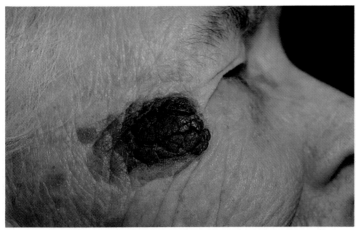

A

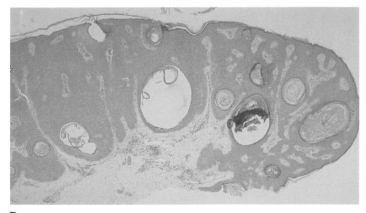

B

4.64
A, Seborrheic keratosis. *B*, Histopathologic appearance of a typical case of seborrheic keratosis.

4.65
Blue rubber bleb nevus syndrome. This autosomal dominant disorder combines cutaneous hemangiomas with gastrointestinal hemangiomas.

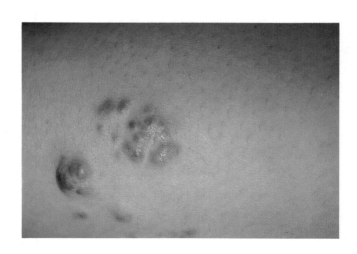

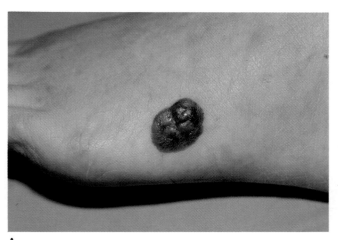

A

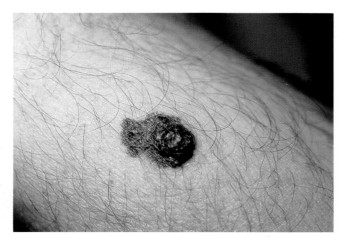

B

4.66
A to *C,* Nodular malignant melanoma. In *C,* note the ulcerated surface in which the surrounding skin has the appearance of superficial spreading malignant melanoma.

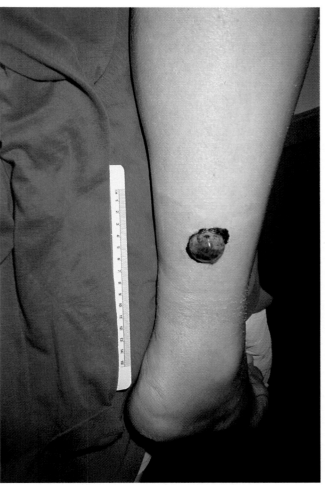

C

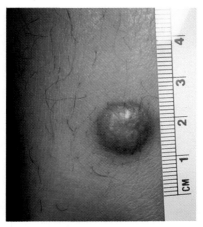

4.67
Dermatofibroma.

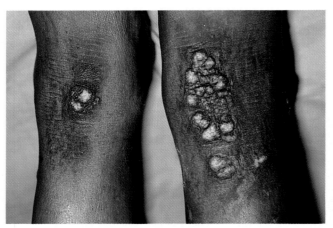

4.70
Prurigo nodularis.

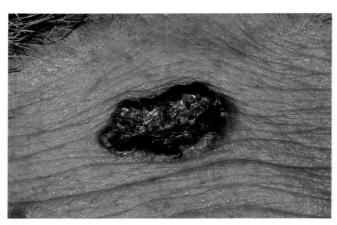

4.68
Pigmented basal cell epithelioma.

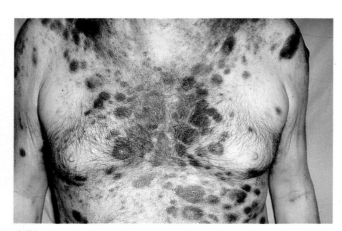

4.71
Cutaneous T-cell lymphoma.

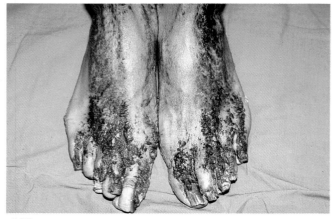

4.69
Epidermal nevus.

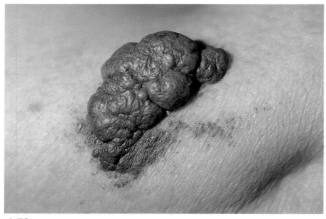

4.72
Capillary-lymphatic malformation (hemolymphangioma).

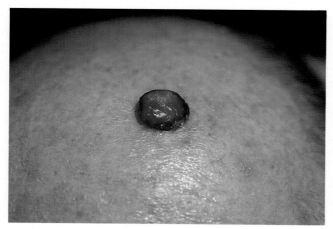

4.73
Atypical fibroxanthoma.

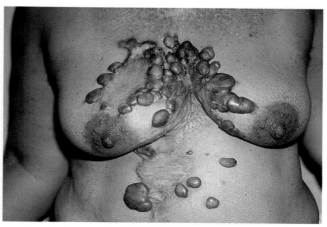

4.74
Keloids.

YELLOW, WHITE, OR CLEAR NODULES

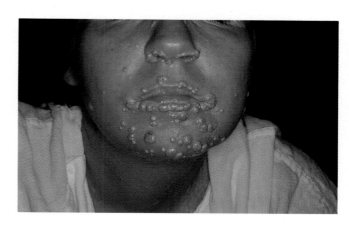

4.75
Eruptive and tuberous xanthomas on a background of hyperpigmented skin. This patient has primary biliary cirrhosis.

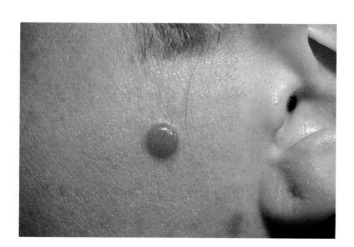

4.76
Juvenile xanthogranuloma. Erythematous orange nodule. This lesion is one that usually resolves spontaneously during childhood.

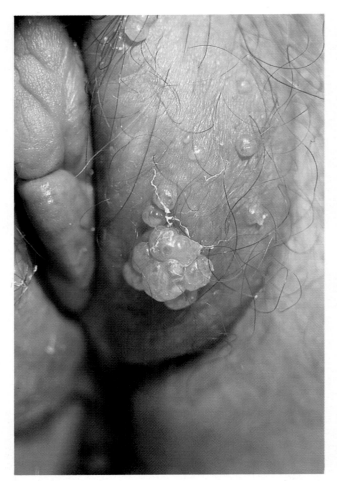

4.77
Lymphangioma circumscriptum, a lymphatic malformation.

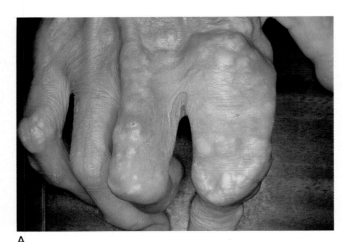

A

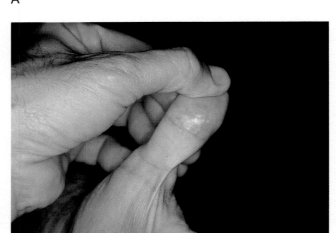

B
4.79
A, B, Tophaceous gout.

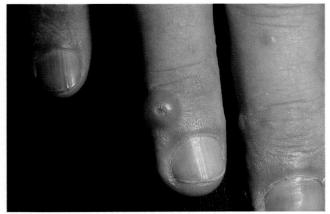

4.78
Myxoid cyst or mucinous pseudocyst.

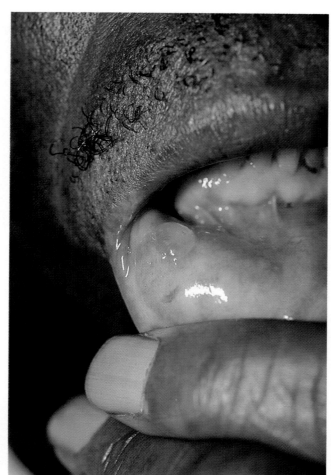

4.80
Mucocele.

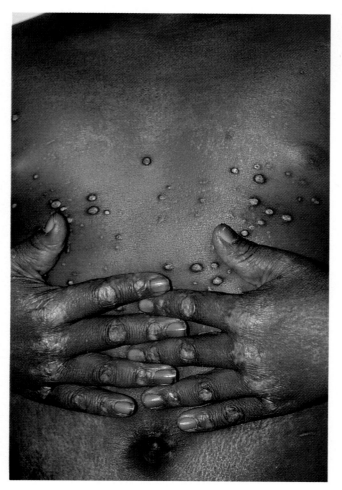

4.81
Calcinosis cutis in a patient with dermatomyositis.

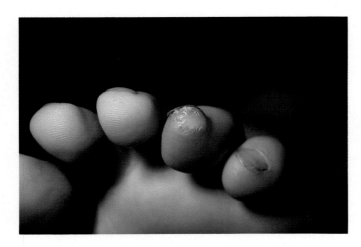

4.82
Osteochondroma.

VESICLES AND BULLAE

These are fluid-containing lesions. Vesicles and bullous lesions represent the primary process that can result in the secondary changes of pustule formation, erosion, and/or ulceration. Histopathologically, these diseases can be divided into those in which the blister is formed within the epidermis (Table III) and those in which the blister is below the epidermis or subepidermal (Table IV). There is also a group of disorders that are inherited and in which the bullae form after trauma to the skin. These disorders are collectively known as the mechanobullous dermatoses or epidermolysis bullosa (Table V). The disorders listed in Tables III, IV, and V can be found in this chapter as well as in the subsequent chapters on pustules and erosions.

TABLE III
Differential Diagnosis of Intraepidermal Vesicles and Pustules

Location of Blister	Disorder
Intracorneal or subcorneal	Staphylococcal scalded skin syndrome
	Toxic shock syndrome
	Impetigo
	Candidiasis
	Subcorneal pustular dermatosis
	Transient pustular melanosis of infancy
	Pemphigus foliaceus or erythematosus
Intraepidermal	Eczematous dermatoses
	Epidermolysis bullosa simplex group
	Friction blisters
	Herpes virus infections
	Incontinentia pigmenti
	Erythema toxicum
Suprabasilar	Pemphigus vulgaris and vegetans
	Hailey-Hailey disease (chronic benign familial pemphigus)
	Darier's disease (keratosis follicularis)
	Transient acantholytic dermatosis (Grover's disease)

TABLE IV
Differential Diagnosis of Subepidermal Blisters

Inflammation	Intact Blister Roof	Dyskeratosis/Necrosis Present
None/sparse	Porphyria cutanea tarda Variegate porphyria Epidermolysis bullosa: junctional, dystrophic, or acquired variants Bullous pemphigoid Amyloidosis	Toxic epidermal necrolysis Acute radiodermatitis Burn Pressure necrosis (coma or surgery)
Predominantly lymphocytes	Lichen sclerosus et atrophicus Polymorphous light eruption Lupus erythematosus	Erythema multiforme Fixed drug eruption Acute graft-versus-host reaction
Predominantly neutrophils	Dermatitis herpetiformis Lupus erythematosus Linear IgA disease of adults or children (chronic bullous dermatosis of childhood) Epidermolysis bullosa acquisita	Septic emboli Leukocytoclastic vasculitis
Predominantly eosinophils	Bullous pemphigoid Herpes gestationis Bullous drug reaction	Arthropod bite reaction
Predominantly mast cells	Urticaria pigmentosa	

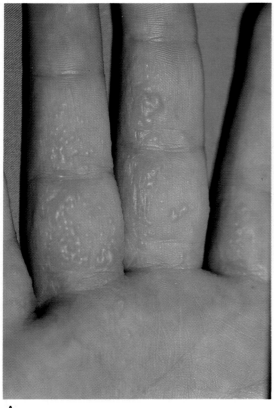

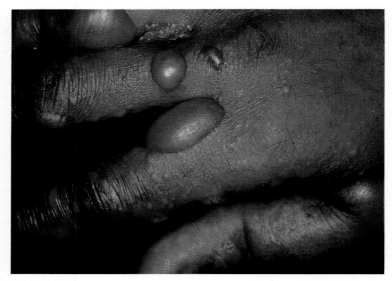

B

5.1

A, B, Dyshidrotic hand eczema. Early lesions show clinical evidence of subcorneal vesiculation, described as a tapioca pudding–like lesion *(A).* With a severe acute flare, the lesions can become bullous *(B)* and are known as pompholyx.

A

TABLE V
Characteristics of More Common Forms of Epidermolysis Bullosa (EB)

Type	Inheritance	Ultrastructural Changes	Features	Other
EB simplex Koebner	AD	Split through basal cells No scarring	Blisters may be generalized	Aggravated by heat
EB simplex Dowling-Meara	AD	Split through basal cells Clumped tonofilaments	Generalized blistering; small, group blisters when older Nail sloughing, thickening; milia as neonate	Defect in keratin 14 gene Aggravated by heat
EB simplex Weber-Cockayne	AD	Split mostly through basal cells	Blisters primarily on hands and feet Nonscarring	Onset may be delayed Aggravated by heat
Junctional EB Herlitz	AR	Split through lamina lucida Reduced hemidesmosomes Absent anchoring filaments	Generalized blisters heal with atrophy Mucosal lesions Nail, tooth involvement	Usually early death Anemia Retarded growth Pyloric atresia
Junctional EB Generalized atrophic benign	AR	Split through lamina lucida May have reduction of hemidesmosomes, anchoring filaments	Generalized blisters heal with atrophy Mucosal lesions Tooth, nail involvement Sparse hair in adults	Normal life span
Dominant dystrophic	AD	Split through sublamina densa Reduced anchoring fibrils	Blisters, especially on extremities Resultant scarring and milia Minimal mucosal change	Collagen VII defect
Recessive dystrophic	AR	Split through sublamina densa Absent anchoring fibrils	Generalized blisters Resultant scarring and milia Mitt deformities Mucosal involvement	Anemia Growth retardation Squamous cell carcinoma Collagen VII defect
Dystrophic inversa	AR	Split through sublamina densa Variable anchoring, fibrils	Blisters at inverse site Milia, scarring Oral erosions, ankyloglossia Esophageal changes, keratitis	

AD, Autosomal dominant; AR, autosomal recessive.

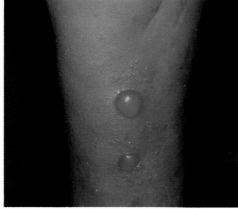

5.2
Bullous stasis dermatitis. Bullous lesions are uncommon in this setting and represent either an acute flare, an infection, or a secondary contact sensitization.

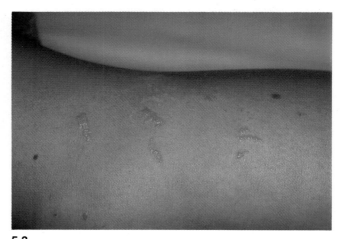

5.3
Contact dermatitis to poison ivy *(Rhus)* results in streaks of vesicles and bullae. The linearity or curvature is suggestive of an external cause.

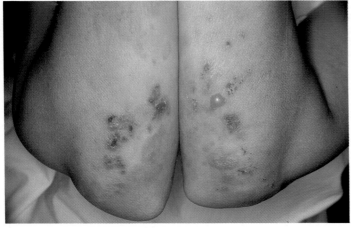

A

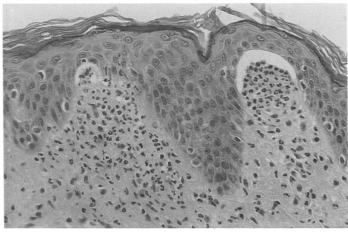

B

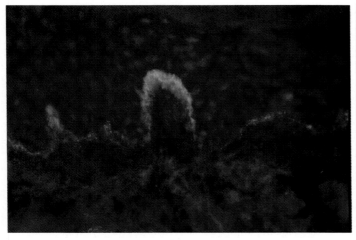

C

5.4
A, Dermatitis herpetiformis (DH) is an immunologically mediated blistering disease. It has a strong association with HLA-B8, DR3. Gluten-sensitive enteropathy is a common associated finding. The lesions are grouped (herpetiform) and extremely pruritic. *B,* Neutrophilic papillitis with subepidermal bulla formation is the typical histopathologic finding in lesions of DH. *C,* Immunofluorescence microscopy of perilesional skin reveals granular IgA deposition in the dermal papillae.

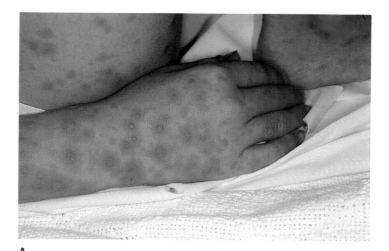

A

5.5

A, Erythema multiforme. Small central vesicles are present on an urticarial base in this child with a viral infection. *B,* Histopathologic appearance of erythema multiforme.

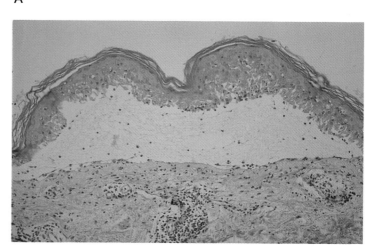

B

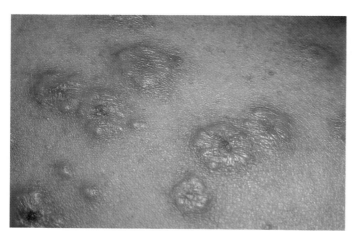

5.6

Bullous leukocytoclastic vasculitis. These lesions are on an urticarial base; often they are on a purpuric base. This is an unusual manifestation of vasculitis.

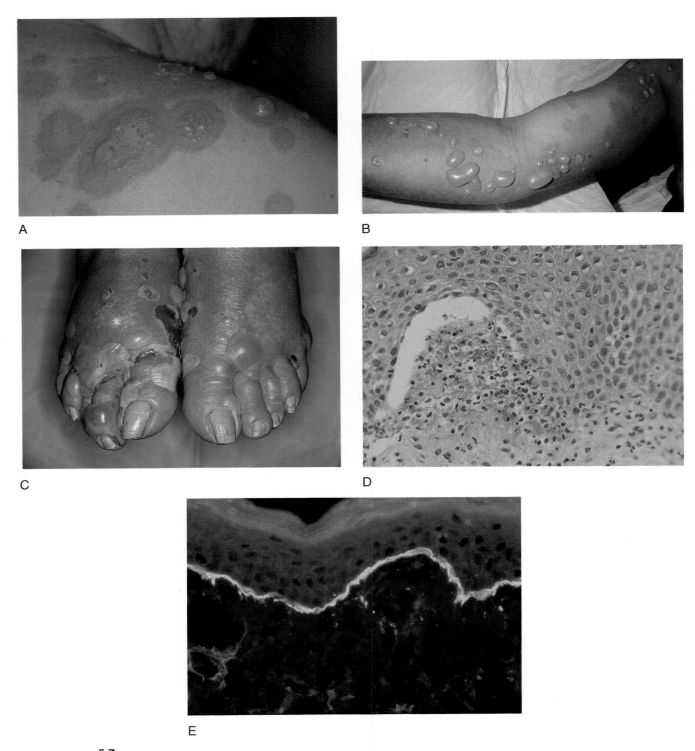

A

B

C

D

E

5.7

A to E, Bullous pemphigoid. The lesions may occur on an urticarial base *(A)* or may be seen without any surrounding erythema *(B)*. With time, pustule formation or erosions can occur *(C²)*. Histopathology reveals a subepidermal bulla with eosinophils in the blister fluid *(D)*. The immunofluorescence pattern is that of linear deposition of IgG along the basement membrane zone *(E)*.

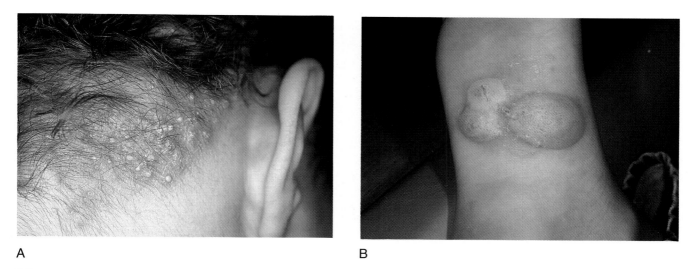

5.8

A, Vesiculopustular reaction to a superficial fungal infection: the kerion of tinea capitis. *B,* Bullous tinea pedis due to *Trichophyton mentagrophytes.*

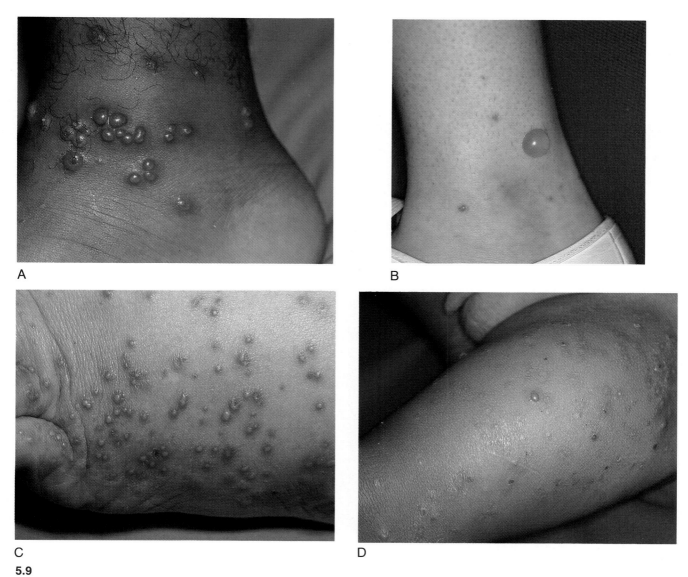

5.9

A to *D,* Bullous insect bite reactions. Flea bites *(A)*, mosquito bites *(B)*, fire ant bites *(C)*, and scabies *(D)*.

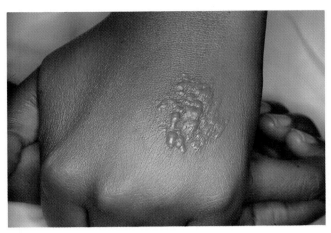

5.10
Bullous fixed drug eruption due to a sulfonamide.

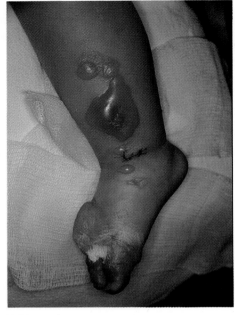

5.11
Chemical burn from an accidental spill.[6]

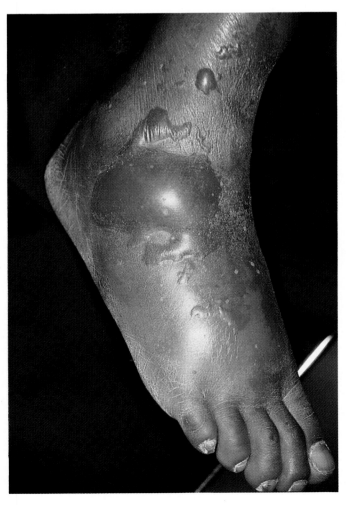

5.12
Pressure-induced bulla.[6]

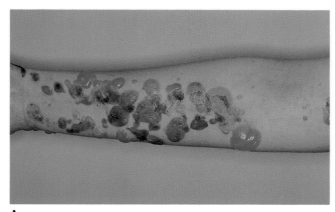

A

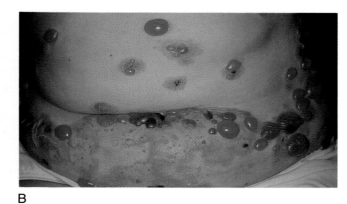

B

5.13

A, B, Herpes gestationis. An autoimmune vesiculobullous disorder associated with pregnancy. The bulla is formed in a subepidermal location and IgG and C3 are found in a linear pattern along the basement membrane zone. This condition is not infectious; the term "herpes" refers to the grouping of the lesions seen in both illustrations.

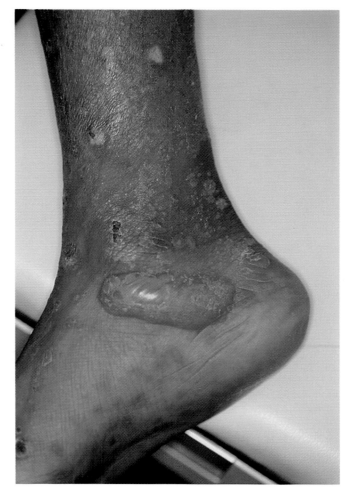

5.14
Bullous lichen planus.

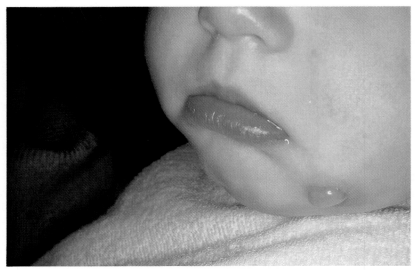

A

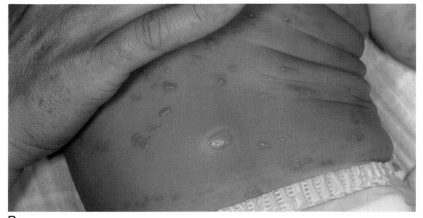

B

5.15
A, B, Bullous mastocytoma (urticaria pigmentosa). This child has had recurrent bullae on the same area of the skin. The bullae develop after stroking the area (Darier's sign).

5.16
Bullous lupus erythematosus. Subepidermal bullae that may histologically simulate dermatitis herpetiformis but immunologically are caused by lupus erythematosus. This process is often associated with active systemic disease.

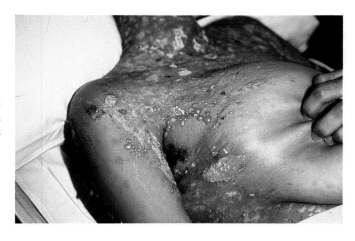

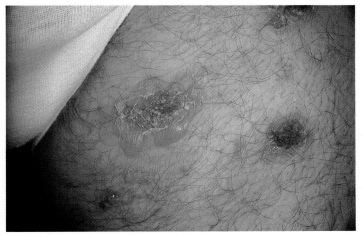

A

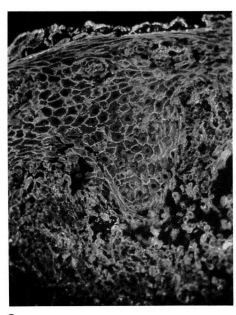

C

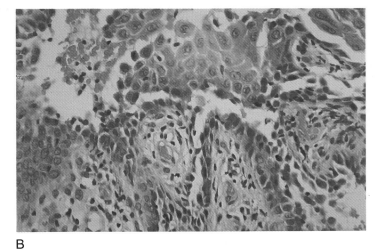

B

5.17

A, Pemphigus vulgaris. Bullae are transient in this disorder; erosion is more characteristic. *B*, Pemphigus vulgaris. The blister is suprabasilar within the epidermis. Individual cells are unattached within the bulla (acantholytic cells). *C*, Deposition of IgG in the intercellular areas of the epidermis is characteristic of pemphigus.

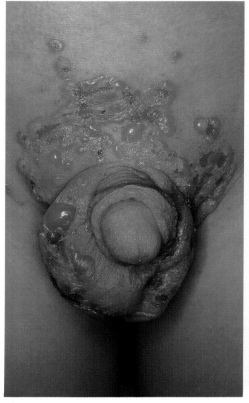

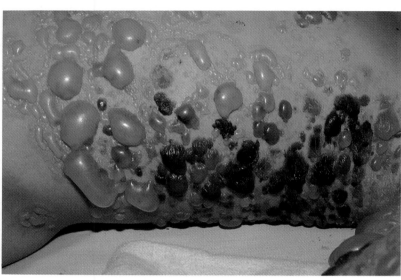

A

B

5.18
A, B, Chronic bullous disease of childhood. This represents a subepidermal bulla with IgA deposited along the basement membrane zone in a linear fashion.

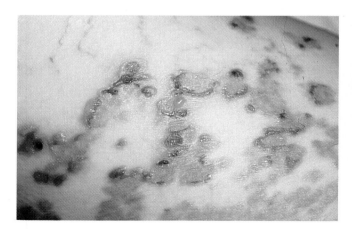

5.19
Linear IgA disease in an adult. The pattern of annular bullae is said to be characteristic of this entity.

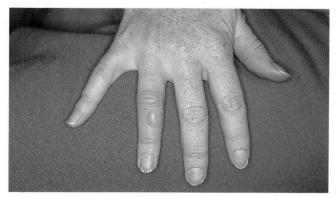

5.20
Phototoxicity from lime juice results in this blister.

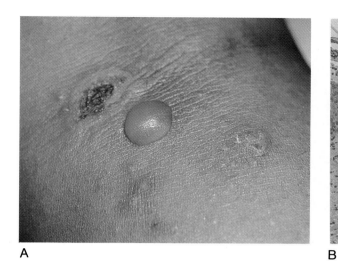

A

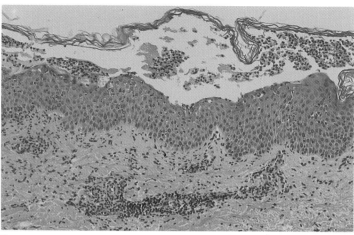

B

5.21
Bullous impetigo. This infection is usually caused by *Staphylococcus aureus*. *B*, Histopathology of impetigo reveals a subcorneal bulla filled with neutrophils.

5.22
Staphylococcal scalded skin syndrome. Due to a toxin produced by *S. aureus* that causes a cleavage in the subcorneal layer of the epidermis.

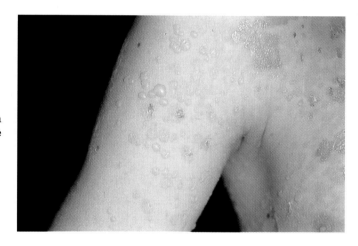

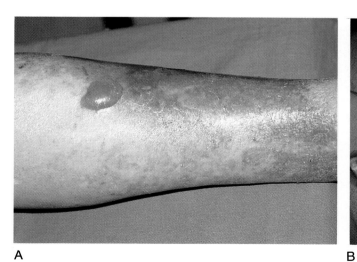

A

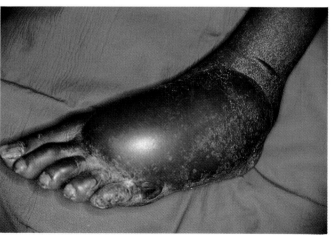

B

5.23
A, B, Diabetic bullae (bullous diabeticorum). Subepidermal noninflammatory bullae in a diabetic patient. (A^5, B^2)

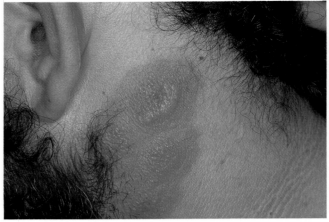

5.24
Bullous lesion in acute febrile neutrophilic dermatosis (Sweet's syndrome).

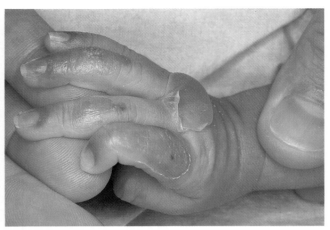

5.27
Epidermolysis bullosa simplex.

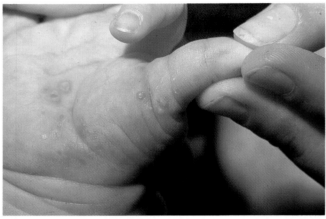

5.25
Acropustulosis of infancy. This process can begin as a vesicular eruption.

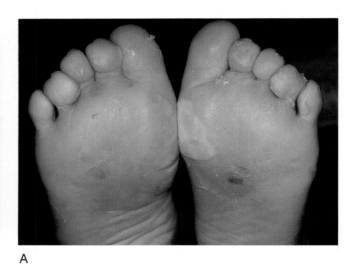

A

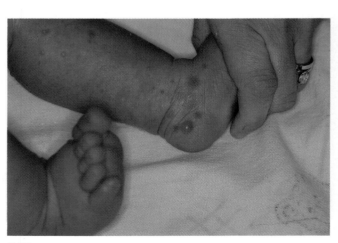

5.26
Transient bullous dermolysis. A benign, self-limited variant of epidermolysis bullosa.

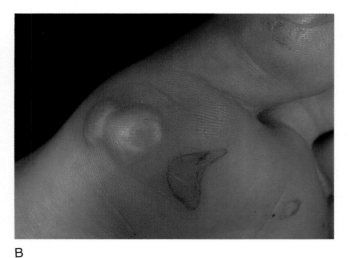

B

5.28
A, B, Weber-Cockayne variant of epidermolysis bullosa simplex.

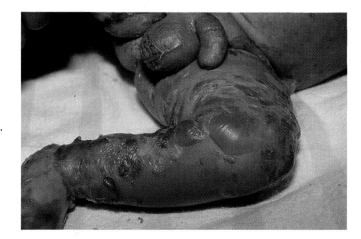

5.29
Dowling-Meara variant of epidermolysis bullosa simplex.

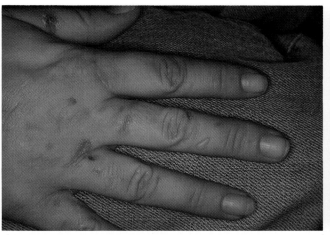

A

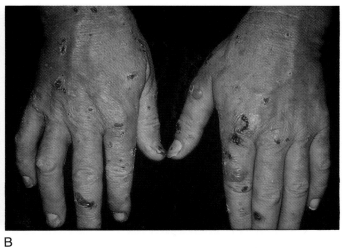

B

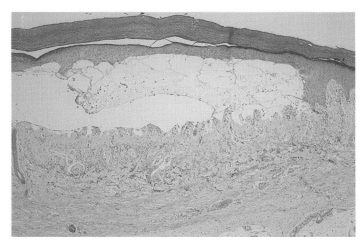

C

5.30
A, B, Porphyria cutanea tarda (PCT). A photoexacer-bated disease. Circulating porphyrins are activated by light and result in energy release, which causes the subepidermal blister to form. Erosions, scars, and milia are also common features of PCT (*A*[4]). *C,* A noninflammatory subepidermal bulla of PCT.

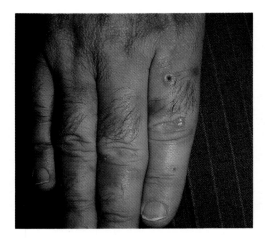

5.31
Bullous dermatosis of hemodialysis. This simulates the changes seen in PCT.

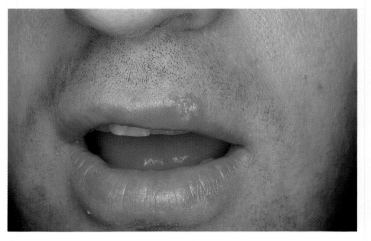

A

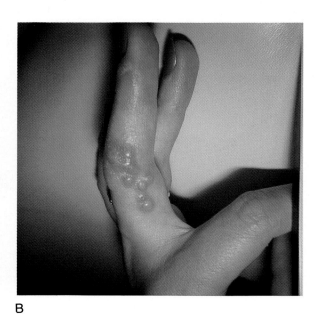

B

5.32
A, Herpes simplex labialis. *B,* Herpetic whitlow: herpes simplex infection of the finger. *C,* Vaginal primary herpes simplex virus (HSV) infection. *D,* Perianal HSV infection. *E,* Recurrent HSV on the thigh. *F,* Histopathologic appearance of HSV reveals an intraepidermal bulla with bizarre multinucleated balloon cells. *G,* A positive Tzanck smear from herpes simplex blister.

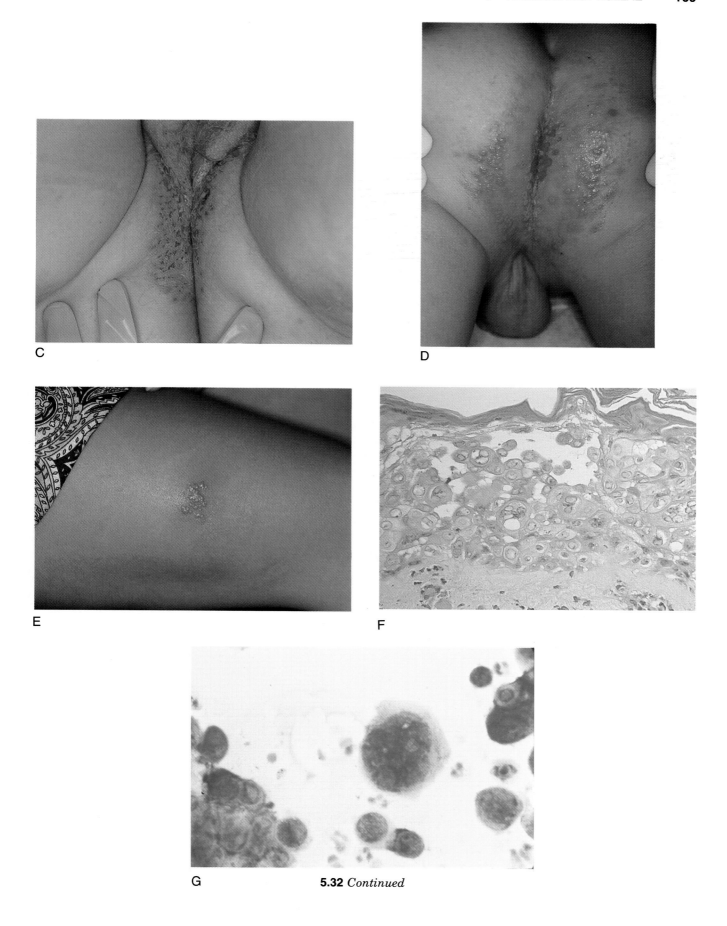

C

D

E

F

G   **5.32** *Continued*

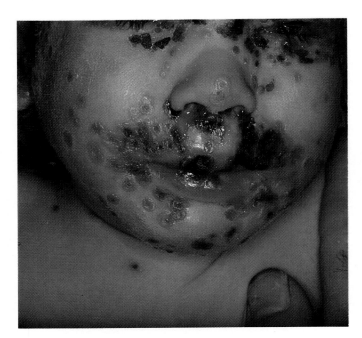

5.33
Eczema herpeticum. HSV infection in a patient with a pre-existing dermatosis, most commonly atopic dermatitis.

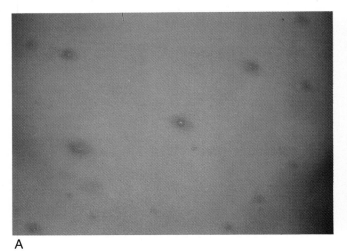

A

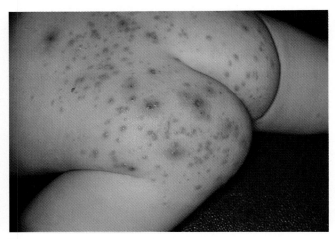

B

5.34
A, B, Varicella (chickenpox). Typical "dewdrop on a rose petal" *(A).* Multiple stages of lesions exist *(B).*

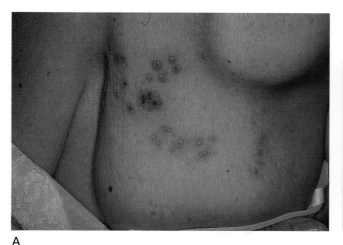

A

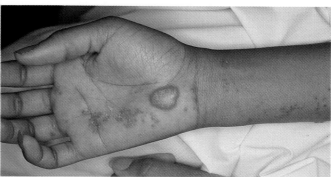

B

5.35
A to *C*, Herpes zoster. This represents a recurrent infection with the varicella-zoster virus. The eruption is usually dermatomal but can become generalized.

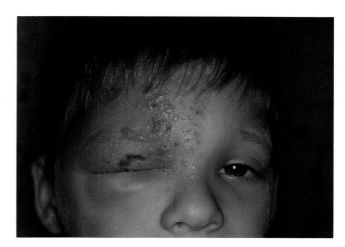

C

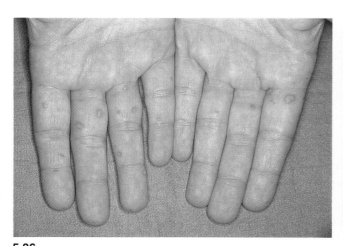

5.36
Hand-foot-and-mouth disease.

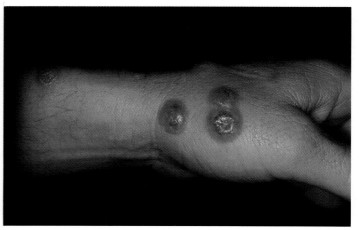

5.37
Cowpox infection. Primary inoculation.

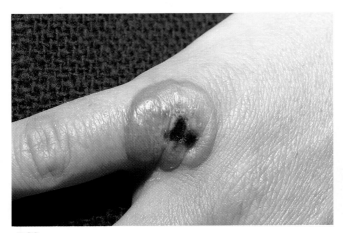

5.38
Orf. Primary inoculation from a sheep or a goat.

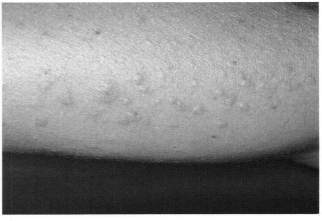

5.39
Polymorphous light eruption, papulovesicular variant.

PUSTULAR LESIONS

Pustules are fluid-filled lesions that contain white blood cells and other debris. Pustules are not always infectious, but a high percentage of the time there is a related infection.

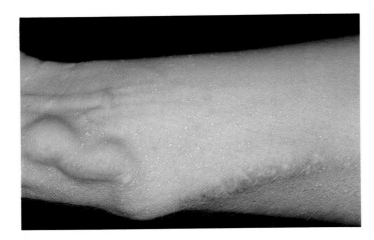

6.1
Miliaria crystallina (heat rash).

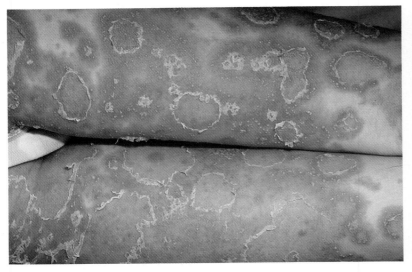

A

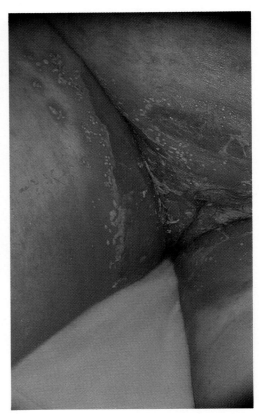

B

6.2
Pustular psoriasis. *A*, Small pustules on an erythematous base with exfoliation of a fine scale. *B*, Sheets of small pustules on an erythematous base.

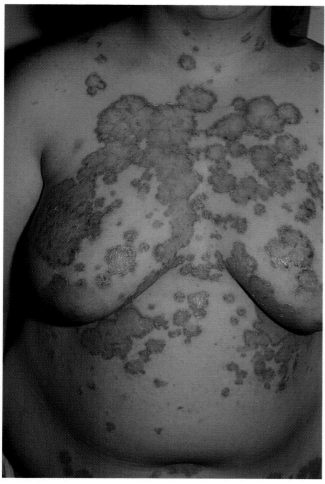

6.3
Subcorneal pustular dermatosis. Pustules stud the periphery of the eroded lesion.

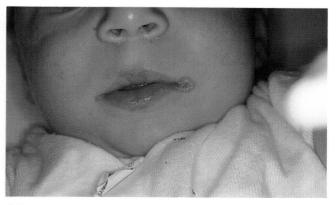

6.5
Acrodermatitis enteropathica. Periorificial pustules are present in this autosomal recessive disorder. Patients have diarrhea, diffuse alopecia, and dermatitis due to an inability to absorb sufficient zinc.[6]

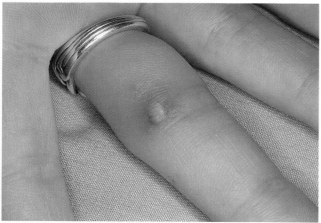

6.4
Disseminated gonorrhea. Pustule on a hemorrhagic base. The typical patient presents with fever, arthritis, and scattered lesions as shown. Cultures from the lesions are usually negative. The best sources for culture confirmation are the oropharynx, cervix, or rectum.

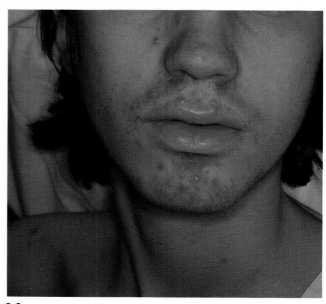

6.6
Acquired zinc deficiency in a patient on hyperalimentation.[3]

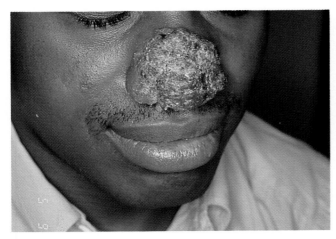

6.7
North American blastomycosis. Verrucous lesion with scattered pustules.

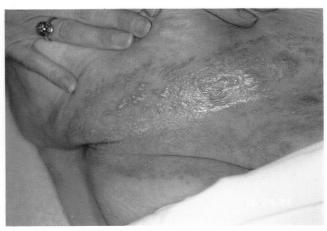

6.8
Candidal intertrigo. Heat and moisture allow an otherwise nonpathogen, *Candida albicans*, to invade the skin.

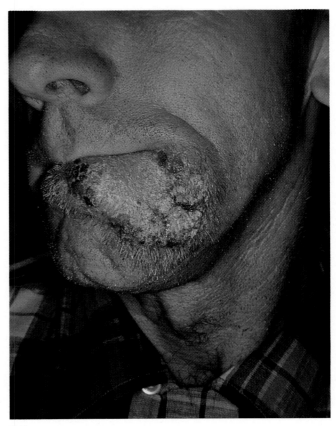

6.9
Tinea barbae due to *Trichophyton verrucosum* infection acquired from handling meat.

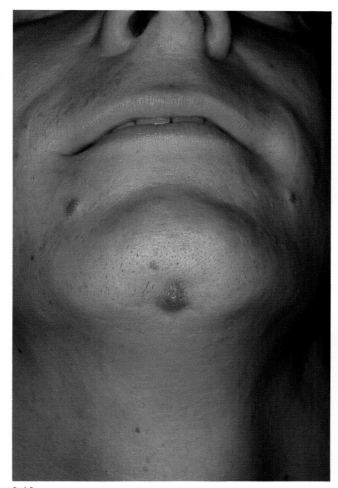

6.10
Periapical abscess due to actinomycosis.

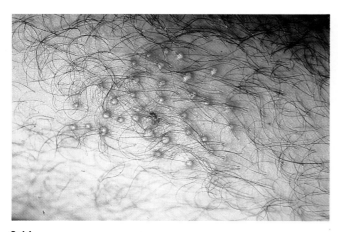

6.11
Folliculitis. Note that the pustules are all follicular. This is usually due to *Staphylococcus aureus*.

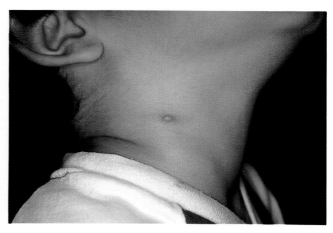

6.12
Cat-scratch disease.

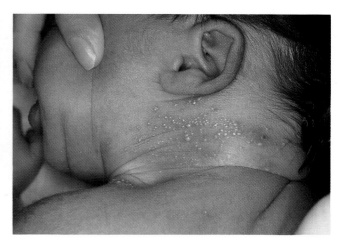

A

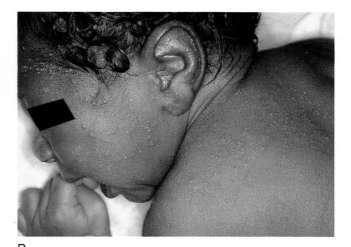

B

6.13
A, B, Transient pustular melanosis. A benign neonatal dermatosis.[2]

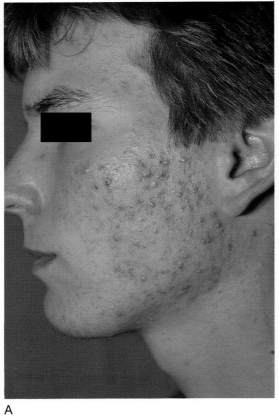

A

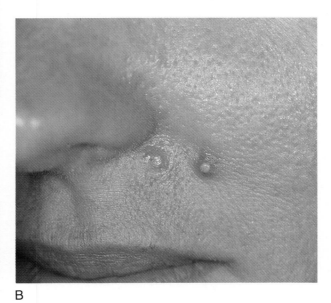

B

6.14
A to *C*, Acne vulgaris.

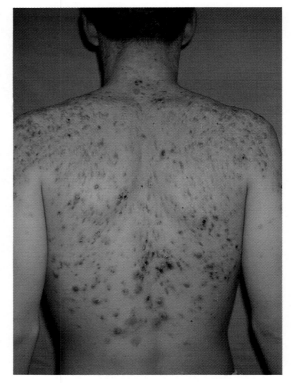

C

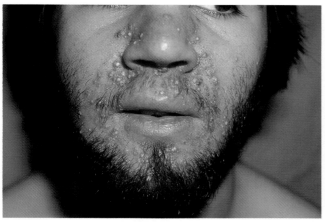

6.15
Gram-negative folliculitis in an acne patient on long-standing antibiotic therapy.

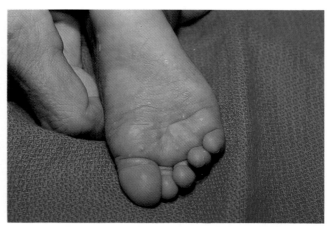

6.17
Acropustulosis of infancy.

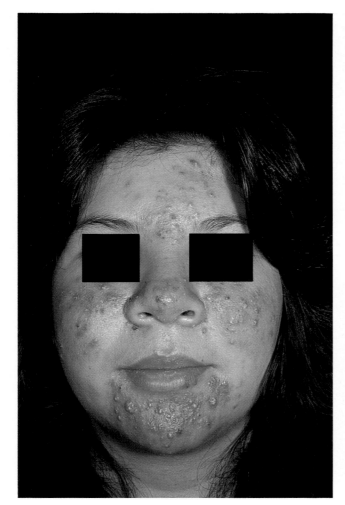

6.16
Acne rosacea.

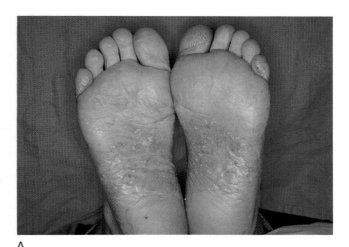

A

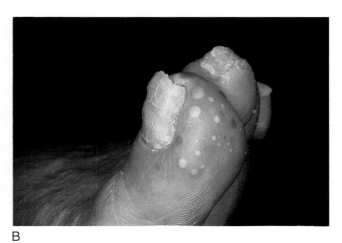

B

6.18
A, B, Pustular psoriasis of the toes and soles.

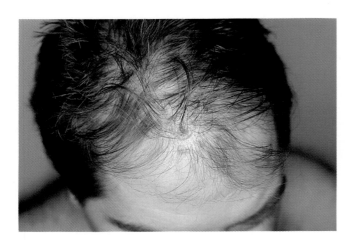

6.19
Vesiculopustular eruption of ulcerative colitis. This patient had an acute onset of fever, vesicles, and pustules in association with a flare-up of the bowel disease.

CHAPTER 7

EROSIONS

Erosions signify the loss of the superficial epidermis. This change usually follows a blister or pustule. Localized erosions due to scratching are termed *excoriations*. Some patients present with severe pruritus, with or without excoriations, in the absence of an identifiable primary cutaneous disease process (Table VI).

TABLE VI
Some Causes of Pruritus (With or Without Excoriations) in the Absence of a Primary Skin Disorder

Delusions of parasitosis
Diabetes mellitus
Drug reactions (e.g., phenothiazines, anabolic hormones, estrogens, progestins, morphine-like compounds, aspirin)
Environmental exposures (e.g., fiberglass, low humidity, obsessive-compulsive bathing, chemical irritants)
Hepatobiliary disease (in particular the biliary tree; e.g., primary biliary cirrhosis)
Lymphoma (in particular Hodgkin's disease)
Parasitic infection
Polycythemia rubra vera
Pregnancy
Psychogenic (e.g., transient emotional stress, obsessive-compulsive behavior, psychoses)
Renal disease (uremia or pruritus of hemodialysis)
Secondary hyperparathyroidism
Thyroid dysfunction (hyper- or hypothyroidism)
Visceral cancer (in particular tumors of central nervous system)

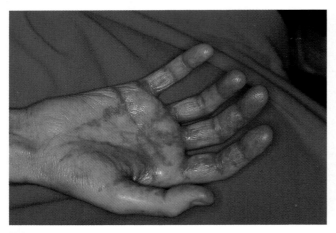

7.1
Candida albicans infection.

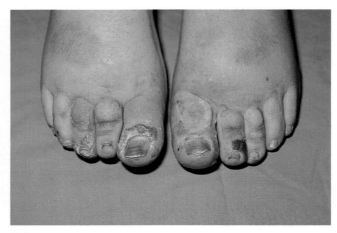

7.4
Epidermolysis bullosa acquisita. An immunologically mediated mechanobullous disease. These patients have antibodies to type VII collagen.

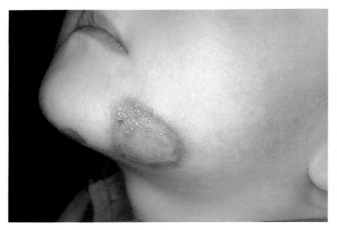

7.2
Tinea faciei.

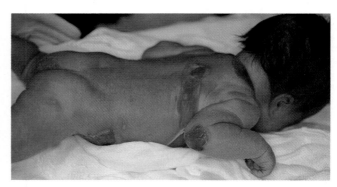

7.5
Junctional epidermolysis bullosa, Herlitz variant.

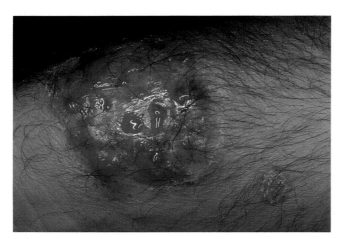

7.3
Kerion. Multiple erosions on the surface of a nodular lesion produced by infection with *Trichophyton verrucosum*.

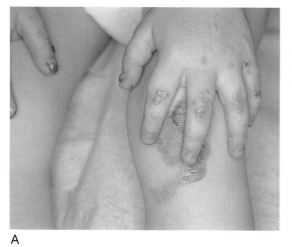

A

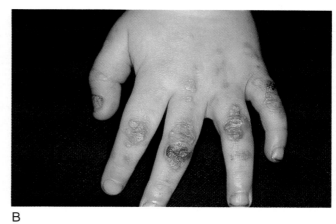

B

7.6
A, B, Dystrophic epidermolysis bullosa, dominant variant.

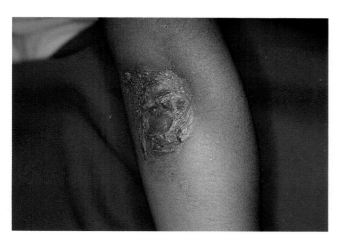

7.7
Generalized atrophic benign epidermolysis bullosa.

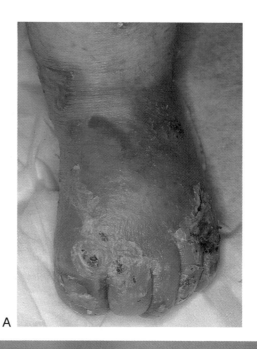

A

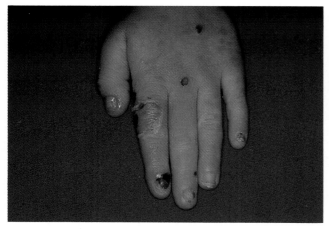

7.8
Dowling-Meara variant of epidermolysis bullosa simplex.

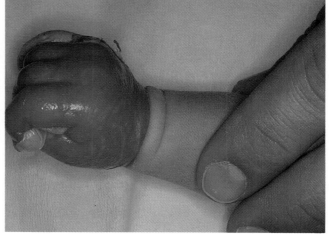

B

7.9
A, B, Recessive dystrophic epidermolysis bullosa.[6]

183

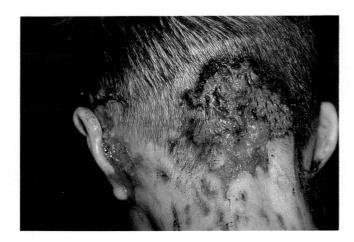

7.10
Localized epidermolysis bullosa dystrophica.

7.11
Inverse recessive dystrophic epidermolysis bullosa. (From Pearson RW, Paller AS: Dermolytic (dystrophic) epidermolysis bullosa inversa. Arch Dermatol 124:545, 1988. Copyright 1988, American Medical Association.)

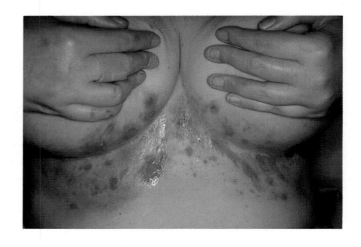

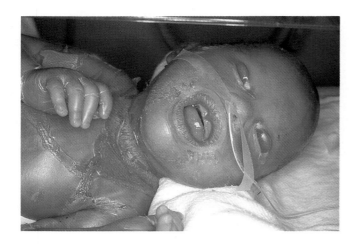

7.12
Collodion baby. Most neonates with this collodion membrane later show nonbullous ichthyosiform erythroderma, but other forms of ichthyosis or even normal skin may follow.

7.13
Porphyria cutanea tarda.

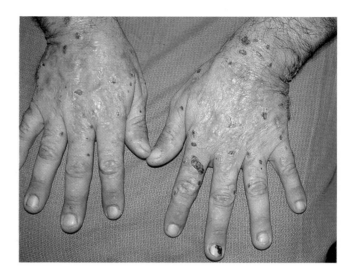

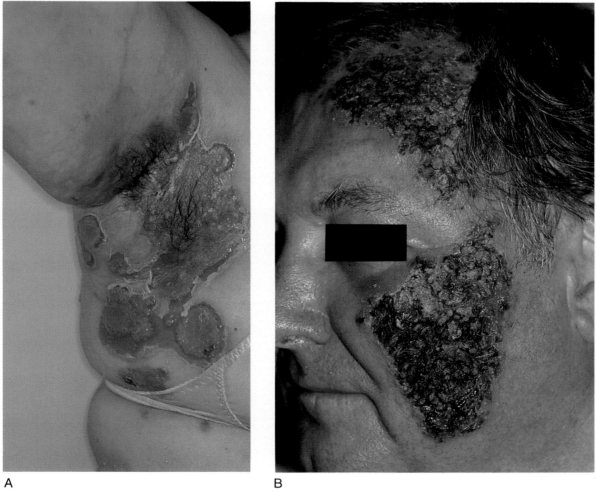

A

B

7.14
A, B, Pemphigus vulgaris. *B,* A vegetative form sometimes called pemphigus vegetans.

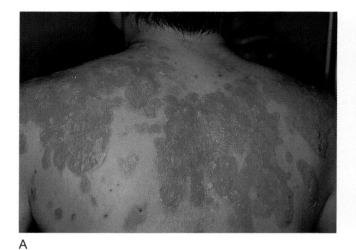

A

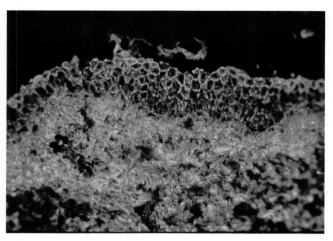

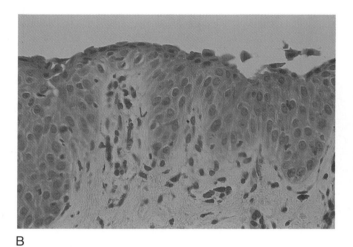

B

7.15

A, Pemphigus foliaceus. A more superficial form of pemphigus in which the split in the epidermis is in a subcorneal location. *B,* Histopathologic appearance of this condition with subcorneal bulla formation and acantholysis. *C,* Immunofluorescence microscopy of pemphigus foliaceus reveals intercellular IgG in the upper epidermis.

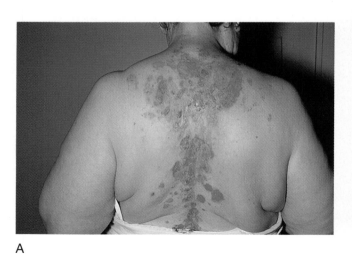

A

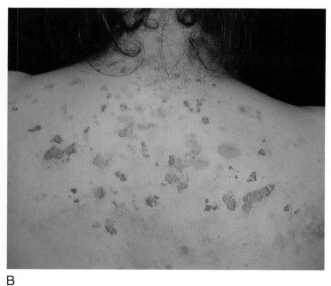

B

7.16

A, B, Pemphigus erythematosus. This combines the immunologic features of pemphigus foliaceus with those of lupus erythematosus. The lesions occur in a photodistribution.

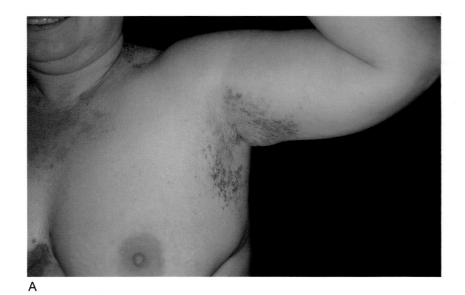

A

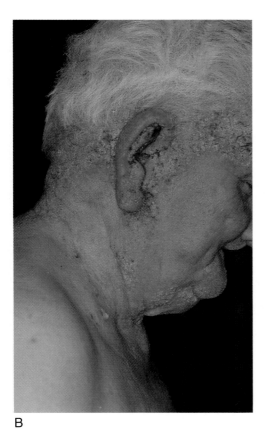

B

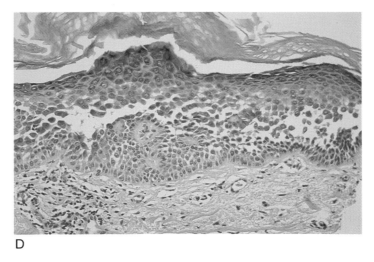

C

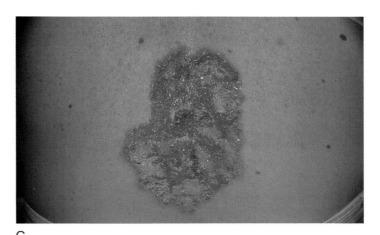

D

7.17

A to *C,* Benign familial chronic pemphigus (Hailey-Hailey disease). An autosomal dominant disorder in which the skin on intertriginous surfaces becomes vesiculated and eroded. Hyperkeratosis and crusting can also occur *(B)*. *D,* Histopathologic appearance of this condition showing dyshesion (acantholysis) of keratinocytes.

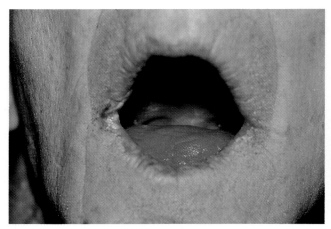

7.18
Perlèche. Erosive dermatitis in the corners of the mouth is a complication of poorly fitting dentures in this patient. *C. albicans* is usually present.[5]

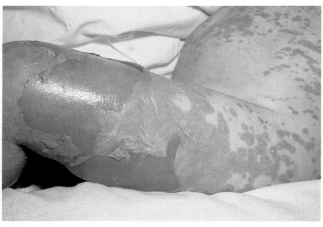

7.19
Toxic epidermal necrolysis. Widespread loss of epidermis with extensive erosions.

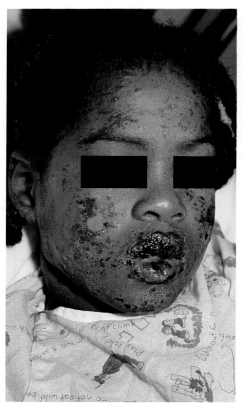

A

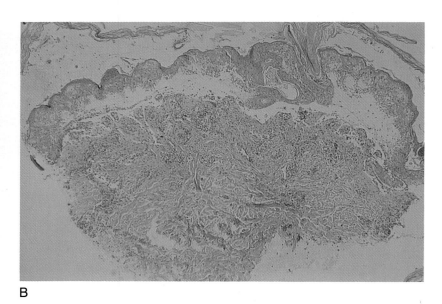

B

7.20
A, Stevens-Johnson syndrome (severe erythema multiforme). Note the extensive oral erosions. *B,* Histopathologic appearance of toxic epidermal necrolysis showing subepidermal separation with a necrotic epidermis.

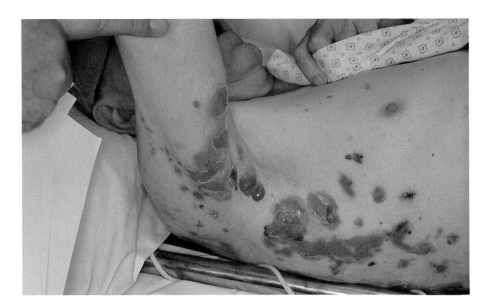

7.21
Bullous pemphigoid. Some intact bullae are seen, but extensive erosions are also present. These lesions heal without scar formation.

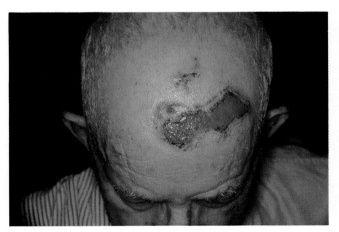

7.22
Brunsting-Perry variant of cicatricial pemphigoid, characterized by extensive erosion and rare intact bullae.

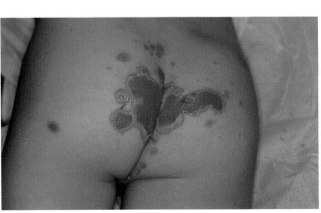

7.23
Chronic bullous disease of childhood. This is the child pictured in Figure 5.18*A* but at a later date. Note the extensive erosive disease.

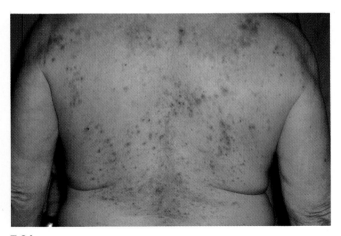

7.24
Transient acantholytic dermatosis (Grover's disease). An acquired condition that presents with pruritic vesicles and erosions on the upper trunk, occurring most often in men.

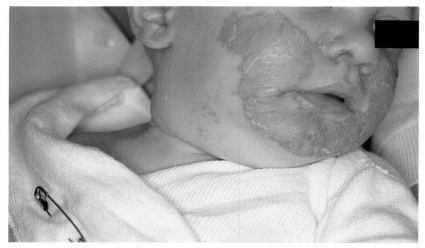

7.25
Acrodermatitis enteropathica. Perioral erosive disease.

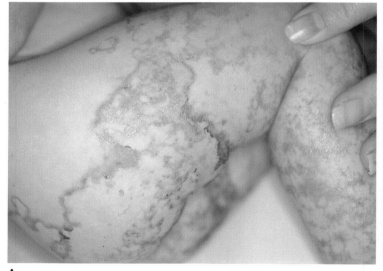

A

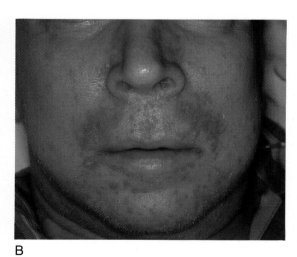

B

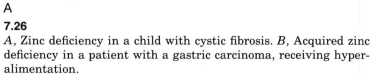

7.26
A, Zinc deficiency in a child with cystic fibrosis. B, Acquired zinc deficiency in a patient with a gastric carcinoma, receiving hyperalimentation.

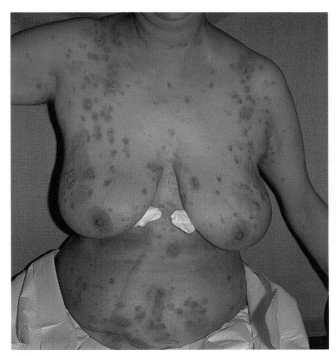

7.27
Subcorneal pustular dermatosis.

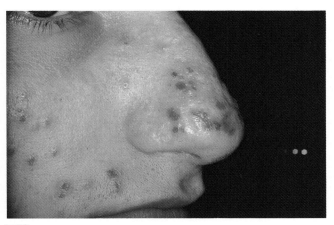

7.29
Hydroa vacciniforme. A severe and bullous variant of polymorphous light eruption. This patient demonstrates erosions following the disruption of the bullae.

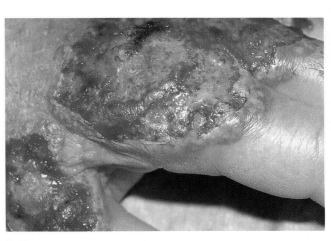

7.28
Atypical pyoderma gangrenosum. An idiopathic inflammatory condition. In "atypical" lesions the process is an erosion rather than an ulceration. The border is a blue-gray bulla that expands. Hematologic malignancy is a common association.

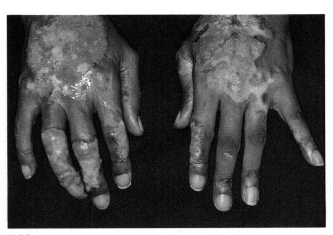

7.30
Discoid lupus erythematosus with extensive erosive changes.

EXCORIATIONS

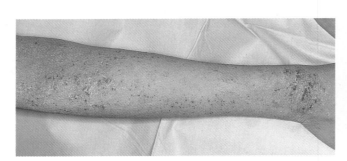

A

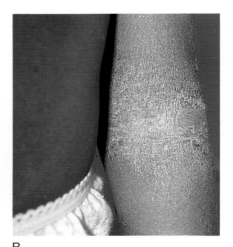

B

7.31

Atopic dermatitis. An extremely pruritic condition. *A,* Multiple excoriations, vesiculation, and marked lichenification are seen in this patient. *B,* Minute excoriations with marked lichenification in the antecubital fossa.

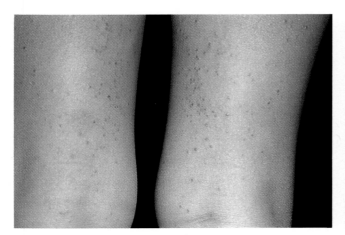

7.32
Papular eczema.

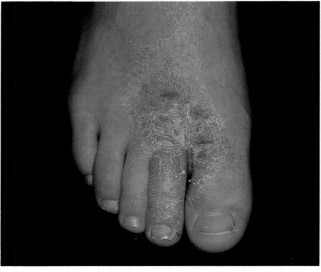

7.33
Chronic eczema of the feet (and hands).

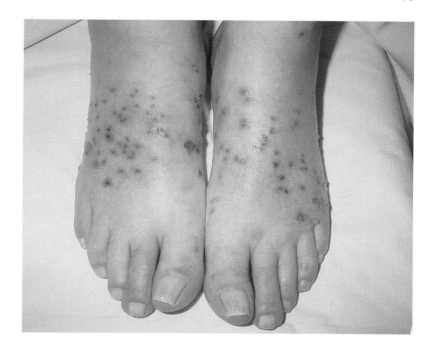

7.34
Insect bites (fleas) led this patient to scratch.

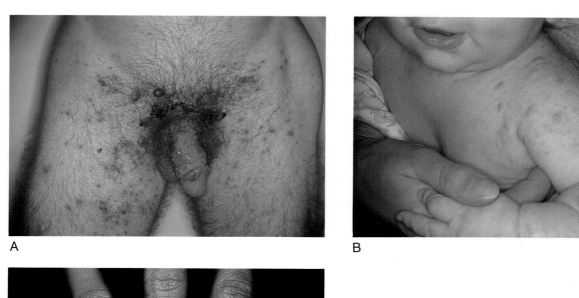

A

B

C

7.35
A to *C*, Scabies. An extremely pruritic infestation (A², C⁴).

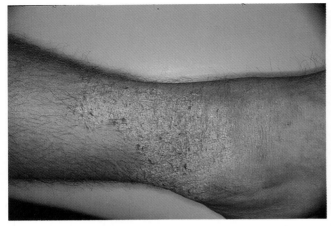

7.36
Lichen simplex chronicus. Patients who chronically rub and scratch their skin can have localized patches.

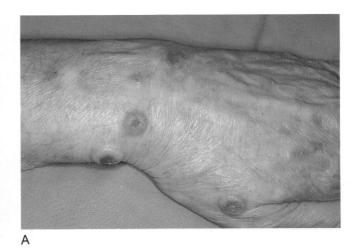

A

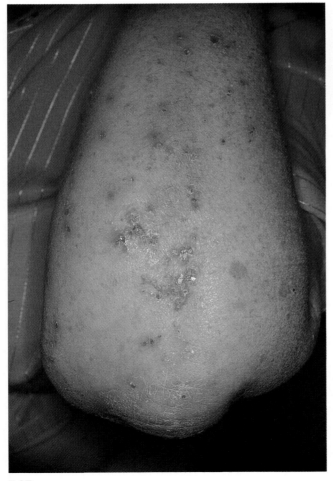

7.37
Neurodermatitis. Multiple excoriations in the absence of a primary skin disease.

B
7.38
A, B, Prurigo nodularis.

CHAPTER 8

ERYTHEMA AND/OR TELANGIECTASIA

Erythema refers to redness of the skin. This is most often due to general dilation of the superficial dermal blood vessels. *Telangiectasia* refers to a localized, often more permanent dilation of the vessels (Table VII). *Poikiloderma* refers to a change that includes dyspigmentation, atrophy, and telangiectasia.

TABLE VII
Differential Diagnosis of Telangiectasia

Primary telangiectasia
  Angioma serpiginosum
  Ataxia-telangiectasia
  Generalized essential telangiectasia
  Hereditary hemorrhagic telangiectasia
  Spider telangiectases
  Unilateral nevoid telangiectasia syndrome
Secondary telangiectasia
  Poikiloderma
  Chronic graft-versus-host disease
  Corticosteroid induced (systemic or topical)
  Dermatomyositis
  Drug induced
  Hepatic cirrhosis
  Lupus erythematosus
  Mastocytosis (telangiectasia macularis eruptiva perstans)
  Bloom's syndrome
  Oral contraceptives
  Pregnancy
  Radiation-induced (x-ray, ultraviolet, or natural sunlight)
  Rosacea, varicose veins
  Systemic sclerosis
  Trauma
  Xeroderma pigmentosum

ERYTHEMAS

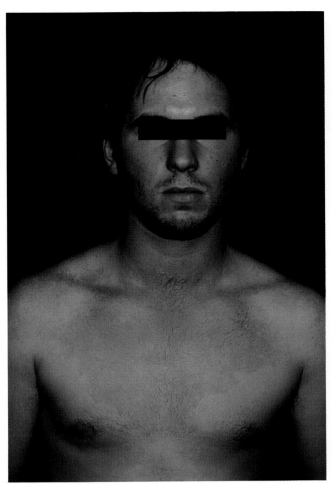

8.1
Flushing in a patient with pheochromocytoma.

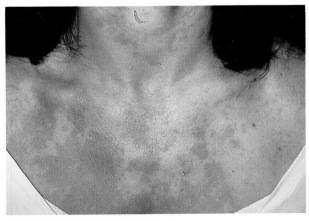

8.2
Flushing due to emotional lability.

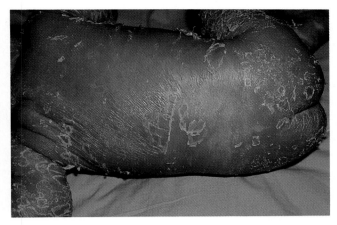

8.3
Pustular psoriasis. These lesions are erythematous with exfoliation and small, sterile pustules.

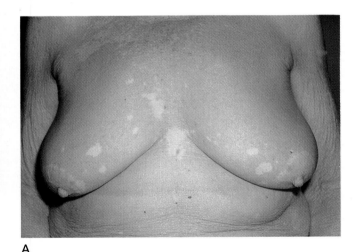

A

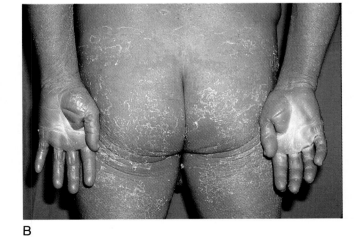

B

8.4
A, B, Pityriasis rubra pilaris. Note the "islands" of normal skin *(A)* and the palmoplantar keratoderma *(B).*

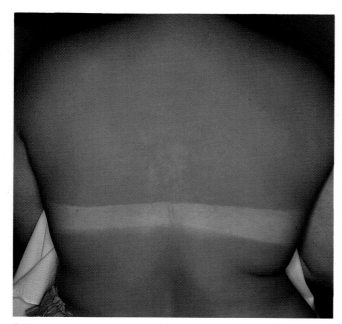

8.5
Sunburn reaction.

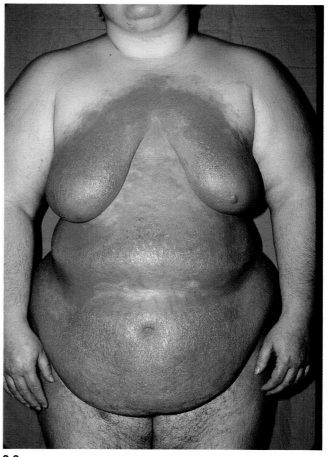

8.6
Irritant contact dermatitis due to the application of anthralin as treatment of psoriasis.

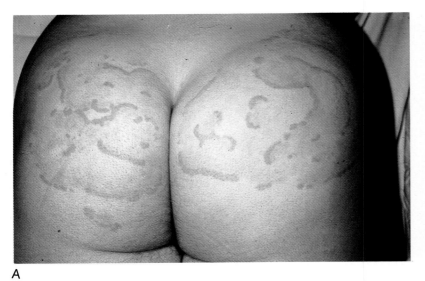

A

8.7
A, B, Erythema annulare centrifugum.

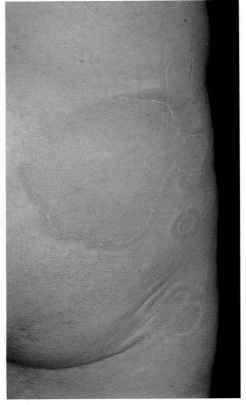

B

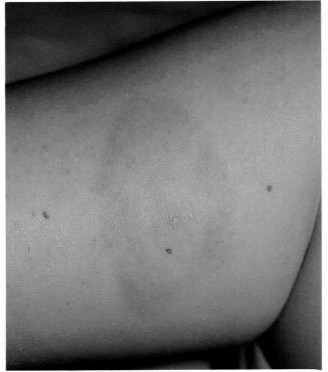

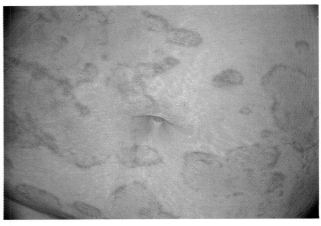

8.9
Erythema perstans.

8.8
Erythema chronicum migrans. A reaction in Lyme disease. Note the central lesion, which was the area of the tick bite.

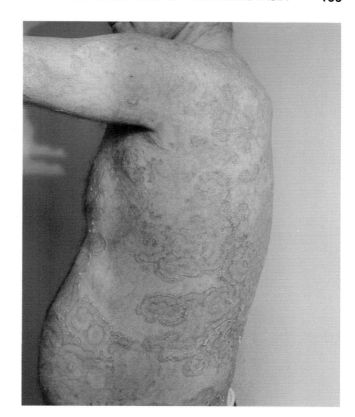

8.10
Pemphigus foliaceus. Annular and serpiginous erythematous lesions.

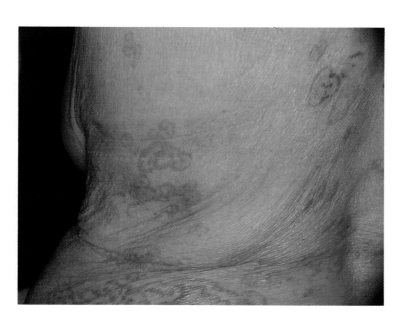

8.11
Erythema gyratum repens. This characteristic lesion is seen almost exclusively in association with internal malignancy.

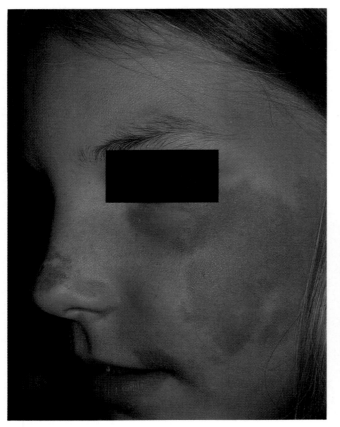

8.12
Nevus flammeus (port-wine stain).

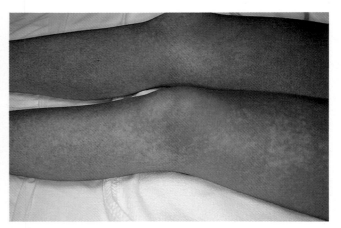

8.13
Toxic shock syndrome.

TELANGIECTASIAS

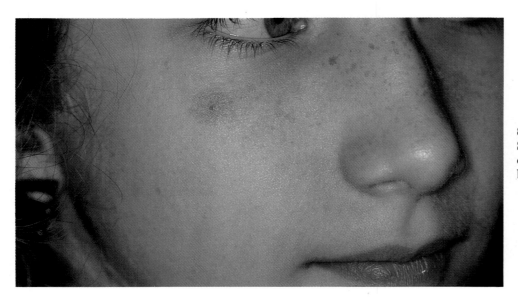

8.14
Spider angioma. There is a central arteriole with a blush at the periphery.

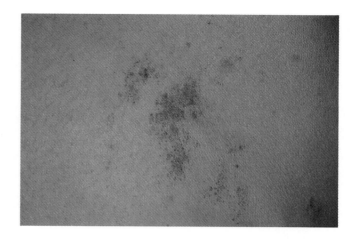

8.15
Angioma serpiginosum. A progressive, localized nevoid condition due to permanent dilation of the superficial dermal vessels.

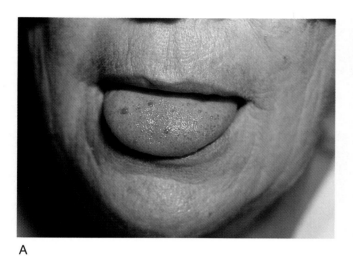

A

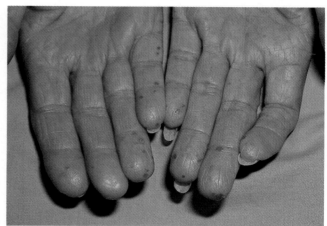

B

8.16
A, B, Hereditary hemorrhagic telangiectasia (Osler-Weber-Rendu disease). An autosomal dominant disorder in which telangiectatic mats are present on the mucosa, lips, and acral areas. There is associated gastrointestinal bleeding, arteriovenous malformations, and epistaxis.

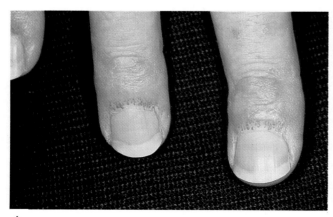

A

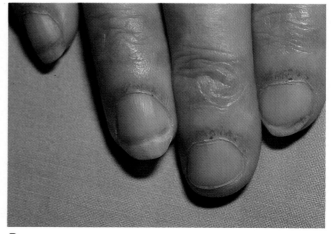

B

8.17
A, B, Periungual telangiectasia in dermatomyositis.

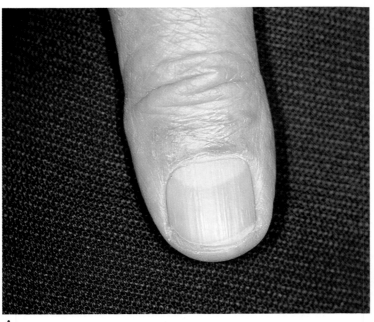

A

8.18
A, B, Periungual telangiectasia in lupus erythematosus *(A)*, telangiectasia in lesions of chronic cutaneous lupus erythematosus *(B)*.

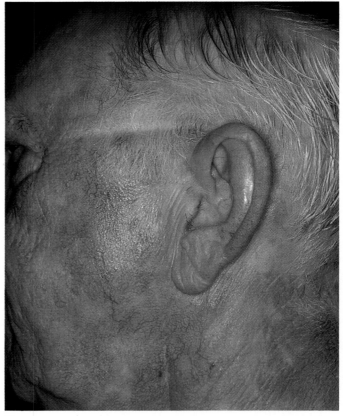

B

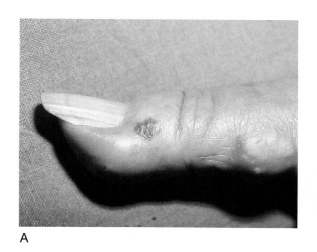

A

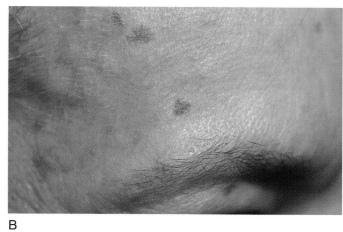

B

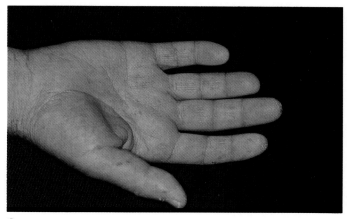

C

8.19
A to *C*, Scleroderma with telangiectatic mats.

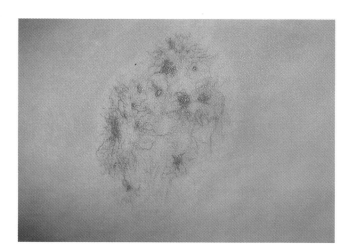

8.20
Essential telangiectasia. This patient has no known underlying disorders.

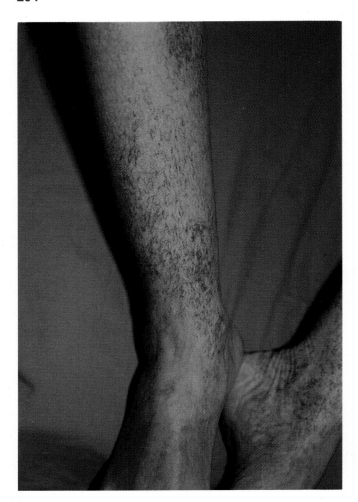

8.21
Generalized essential telangiectasia.

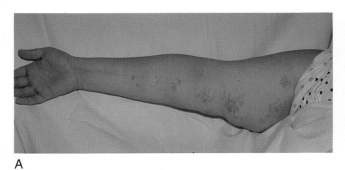

A

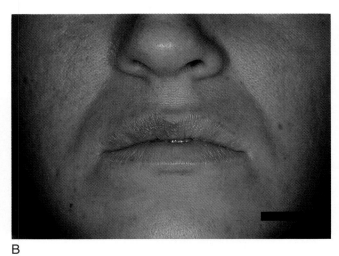

B

8.22
A, B, Unilateral nevoid telangiectasia.

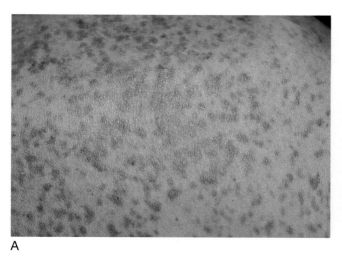

A

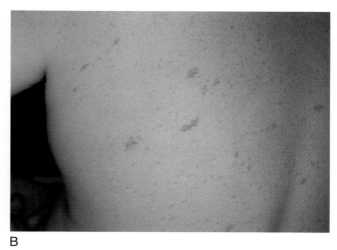

B

8.23

A, B, Telangiectasia macularis eruptiva perstans. A variant of urticaria pigmentosa (mastocytoma of the skin).

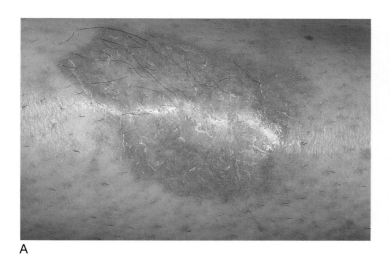

A

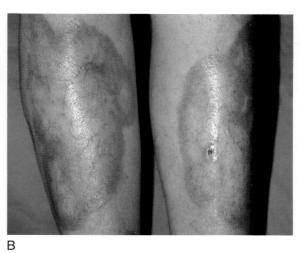

B

8.24

A, B, Telangiectasia in necrobiosis lipoidica diabeticorum.

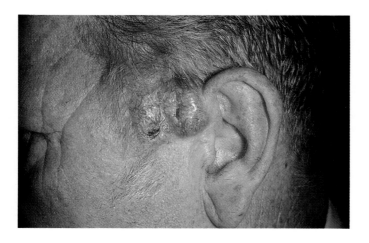

8.25

Prominent telangiectasia in basal cell carcinoma.

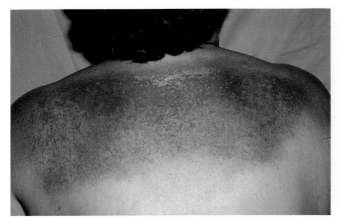

8.26
Acute radiation dermatitis.

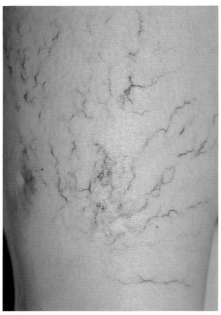

8.27
Starburst of dilated superficial veins.

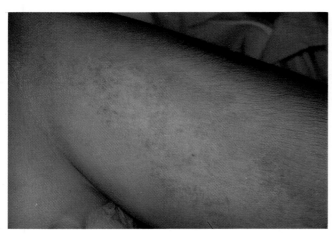

8.28
Poikiloderma in childhood dermatomyositis.

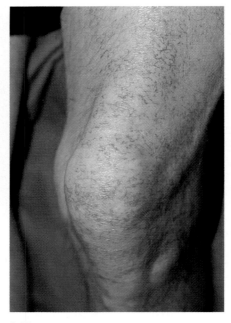

8.29
Werner's syndrome (adult progeria). An autosomal recessive disorder characterized by premature aging (baldness, osteoporosis, cataracts, and atherosclerotic vascular disease), poikiloderma, hypogonadism, and a high-pitched voice.

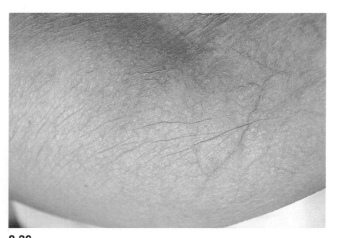

8.30
Telangiectasia in a patient with cutaneous atrophy due to the chronic use of potent topical corticosteroids.

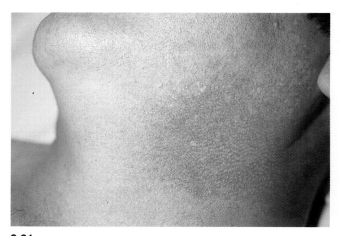

8.31
Poikiloderma of Civatte in a light-exposed area of the neck.

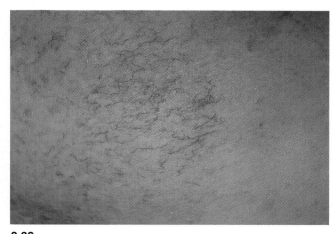

8.33
Chronic radiation dermatitis.

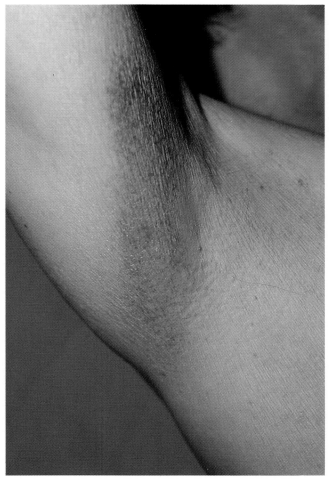

8.32
Poikilodermatous mycosis fungoides.

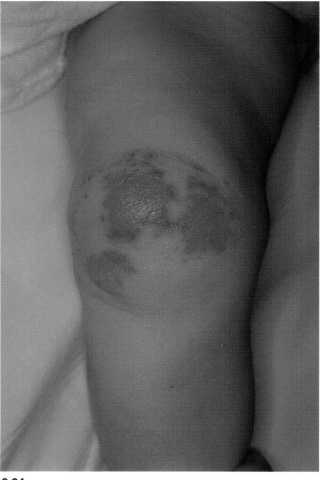

8.34
Acrodermatitis enteropathica.

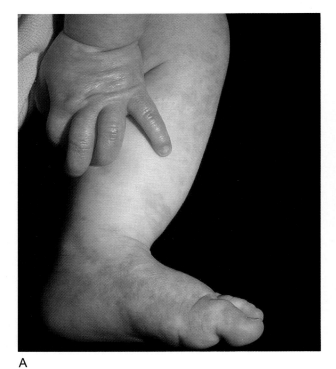

A

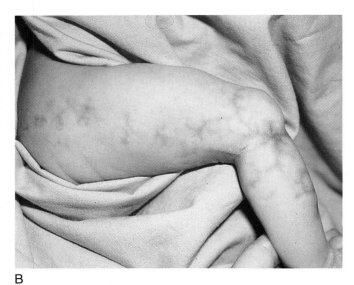

B

8.35
A, B, Cutis marmorata. A reticulated pattern of dilated blood vessels.

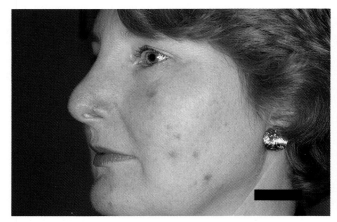

8.36
Sarcoidosis.

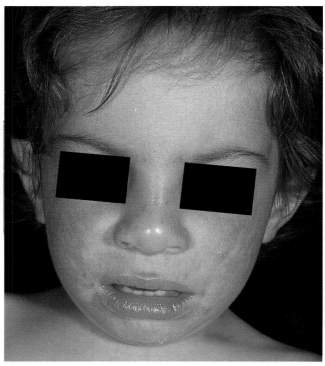

8.37
Bloom's syndrome. This autosomal recessive disorder is characterized by photosensitivity, congenital facial erythema, telangiectasia, and stunted growth.

PURPURA

Purpura results from leakage of blood into the skin or mucous membranes. Purpuras are divided into those that are palpable and those that are nonpalpable. Palpable purpuras suggest an inflammatory (immunologic or infectious) vasculopathy; nonpalpable purpuras occur with trauma or coagulopathy. Purpuras can be described as petechial, which term is reserved for small lesions, or ecchymotic, which refers to larger lesions.

NONPALPABLE PURPURA

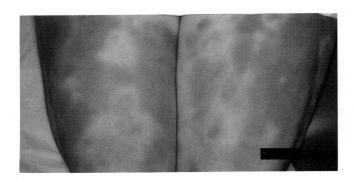

9.1
Gardner-Diamond syndrome (autoerythrocyte sensitization syndrome). This rare disorder occurs almost exclusively in young women. Trauma initiates the purpuric lesion. Patients often have an abnormal psychiatric profile.

9.2
Ehlers-Danlos syndrome, Type IV (ecchymotic variant). This condition shows a variety of patterns of inheritance. It is associated with easy bruising, fragility of the skin, and vascular and/or gastrointestinal rupture.

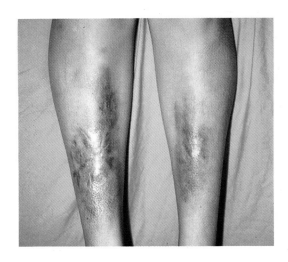

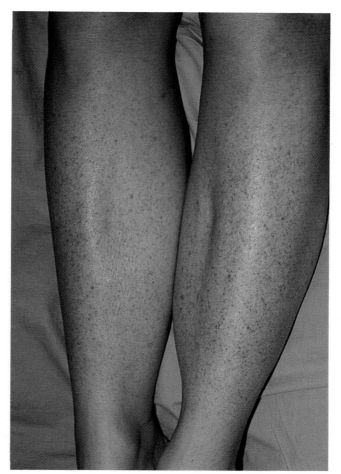

A

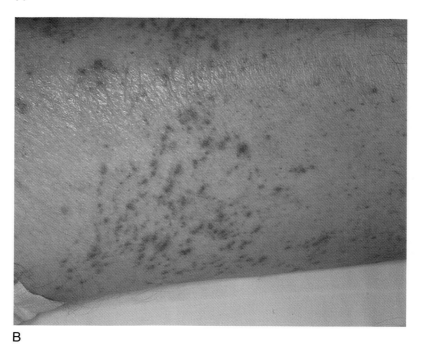

B

9.3

A, Idiopathic thrombocytopenic purpura. Increased platelet destruction due to an immunologic reaction. *B*, Drug-induced thrombocytopenia.

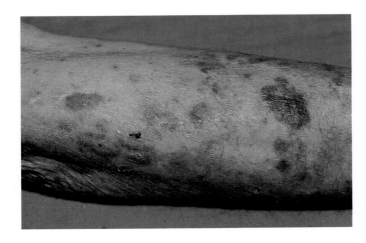

9.4
Corticosteroid-induced purpura.[5]

9.5
"Pinch-purpura" of primary systemic amyloidosis. This patient, like most individuals with primary systemic amyloidosis, had multiple myeloma.

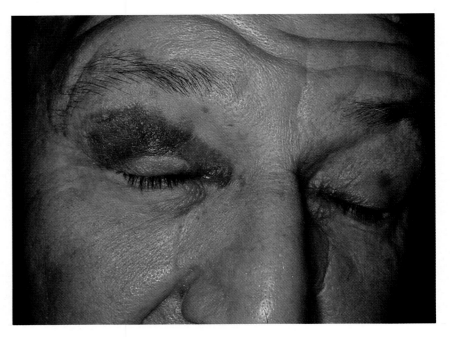

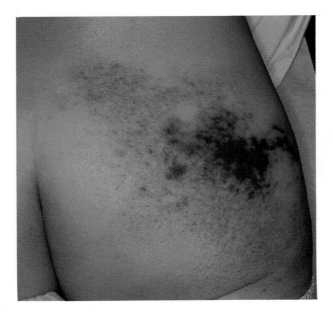

9.6
Cryoglobulinemia.

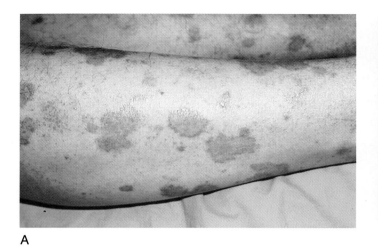

A

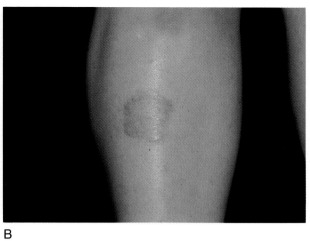

B

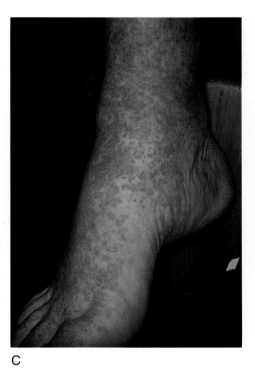

C

9.7
A to *D,* Capillaritis. Purpura annularis telangiectoides (*A,* *B*), Majocchi's disease *(C)*, and Schamberg's disease *(D)*.

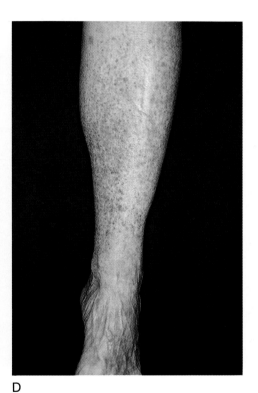

D

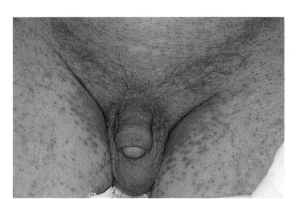

9.8
Scurvy. Vitamin C deficiency results in perifollicular purpura, corkscrew hairs, and folliculitis.

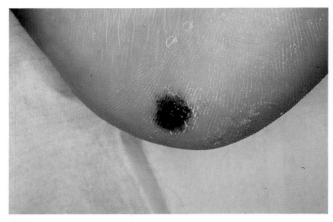

9.9
Talon noir. Hemorrhage into the heel due to athletic trauma.

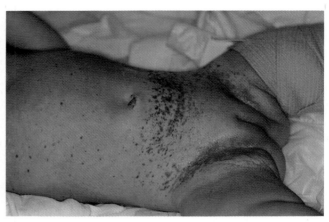

9.10
Purpura of histiocytosis X.

PALPABLE PURPURA

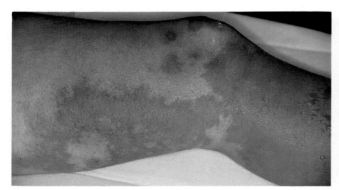

9.11
Disseminated intravascular coagulopathy in a patient with gram-negative sepsis.[2]

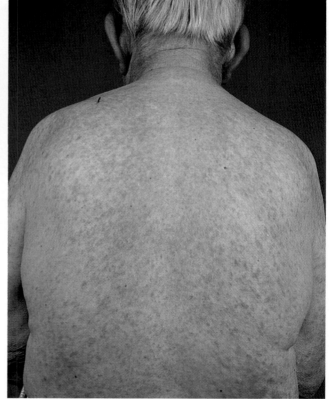

9.12
Angioimmunoblastic lymphadenopathy.[1]

9.13
Acute febrile neutrophilic dermatosis (Sweet's syndrome) in a patient with acute myelogenous leukemia complicated by thrombocytopenia.

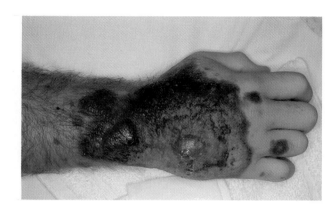

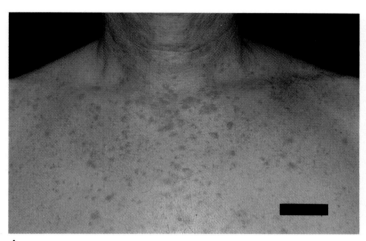

A

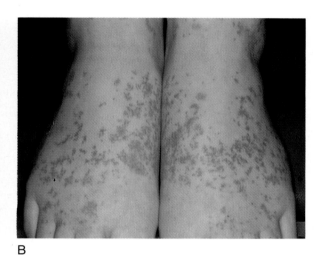

B

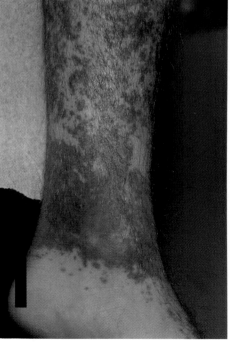

C

9.14
A, Early lesions of leukocytoclastic vasculitis (Table VIII). B, Leukocytoclastic vasculitis due to IgA immune complexes in a patient with IgA nephropathy. C, Drug-induced cutaneous leukocytoclastic vasculitis.

I. Entities manifested by palpable purpura and LCV histopathologically
Idiopathic
Henoch-Schönlein purpura (IgA-related LCV)
  Non-IgA vasculitis
  Acute hemorrhagic edema of infancy
Infectious (any infection can be associated, but the following may be more common)
  Streptococcus   Otitis media
  Hepatitis B   Meningococcemia
  Influenza   Gonococcemia
  Mononucleosis
Systemic disease
  Lupus erythematosus   Sjögren's syndrome
  Rheumatoid arthritis   Scleroderma
  Dermatomyositis   Inflammatory bowel disease
  Chronic active hepatitis Wegener's granulomatosis
  Cryoglobulinemia or other
    paraproteinemia
Malignancy ("paraneoplastic vasculitis")
  Leukemia and lymphoma   Hodgkin's disease
  Multiple myeloma   Solid tumors
Drugs and chemicals (any drug can be associated, but the following are perhaps more common)
  Penicillin   Sulfonamides
  Quinidine   Allopurinol
  Propylthiouracil   Food additives

II. Entities that demonstrate LCV histopathologically but may not exhibit palpable purpura
Hypocomplementemic (urticarial) vasculitides
Degos' disease
Erythema elevatum diutinum

III. Entities that may demonstrate palpable purpura but are not LCV histopathologically
Antiphospholipid antibody syndrome
Embolic phenomenon
  Bacterial endocarditis
  Atheroemboli
  Cholesterol emboli
  Left atrial myxoma
  Purpura fulminans
  Coumarin necrosis
  Disseminated intravascular coagulopathy

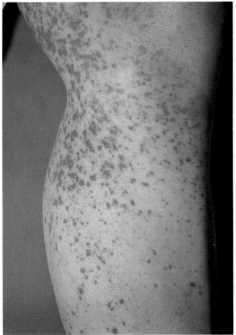

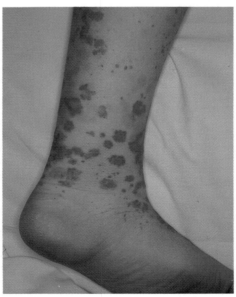

A

B

9.15
A, B, Henoch-Schönlein purpura. This combines palpable purpura, arthritis, and gastrointestinal involvement and occasionally nephritis and central nervous system involvement. The process appears to be related to IgA-containing immune complexes.

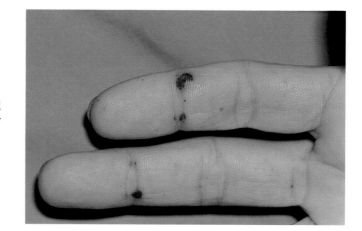

9.16
Patients with Wegener's granulomatosis may have small vessel vasculitis of the skin. This phenomenon is usually accompanied by active systemic disease.

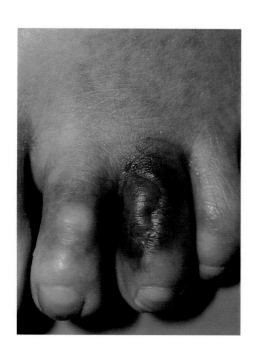

9.17
Purpura due to emboli in a patient with severe atherosclerotic peripheral vascular disease.

9.18
Disseminated lesions in gonococcemia.[2]

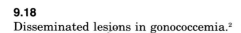

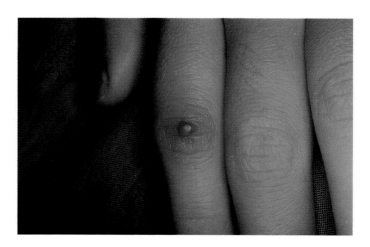

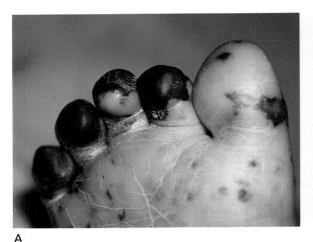

A

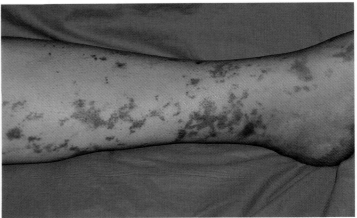

B

9.19
A to *C,* Meningococcemia, a consumptive coagulopathy. Purpura is secondary.

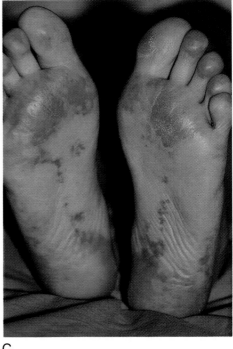

C

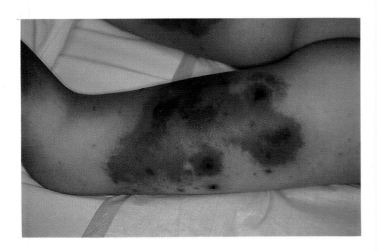

9.20
Purpura fulminans after a varicella infection.

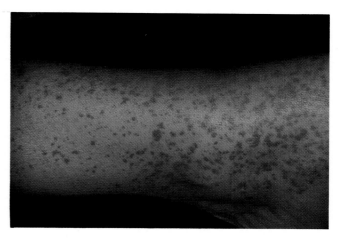

9.21
Hyperglobulinemic purpura. This most likely represents a leukocytoclastic vasculitis in a patient with hyperglobulinemia. Sjögren's syndrome is also frequently found.

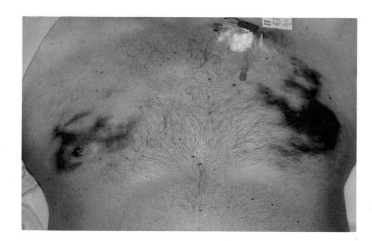

9.22
Cryoglobulinemia.[5]

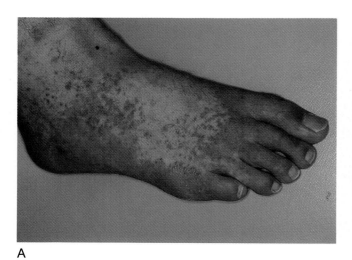

A

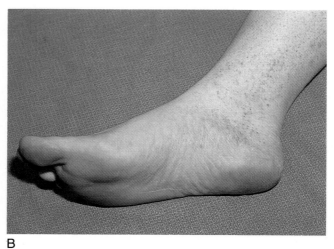

B

9.23
A, B, Petechial eruption of Rocky Mountain spotted fever.

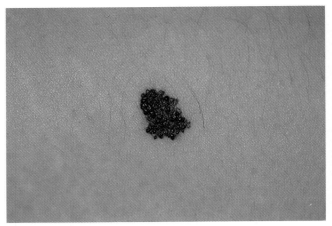

9.24
Angiokeratoma.

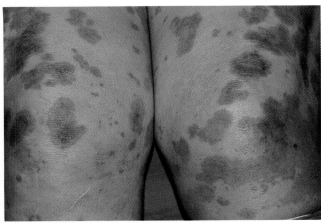

9.26
Erythema elevatum diutinum. This entity is a localized chronic form of cutaneous small vessel vasculitis.

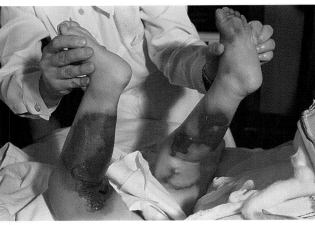

9.27
Acute hemorrhagic edema of infancy. An acute, edematous purpura in infants, usually those under 4 years of age. This process resolves spontaneously and is not associated with severe systemic involvement.

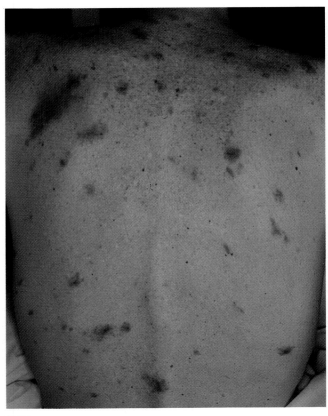

9.25
Kaposi's sarcoma.

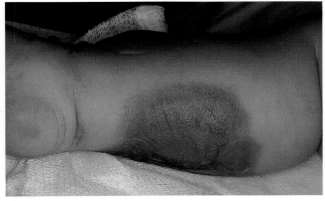

9.28
Chemical burn in a newborn.[6]

10 ULCERS

An ulcer is a lesion with total epidermal loss and partial or total loss of the dermis. When ulcers heal, they heal with a scar.

NONGENITAL ULCERATIONS

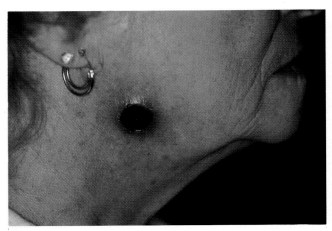

10.1
Persistent bite reaction. This intense reaction resulted in a central ulceration of the nodule.

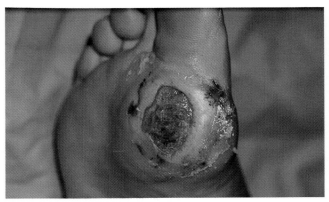

10.2
Neurotropic ulcer in a diabetic patient with peripheral neuropathy.

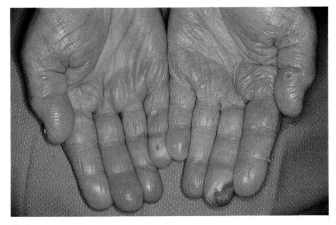

10.3
Lepromatous leprosy with neuropathy.[2]

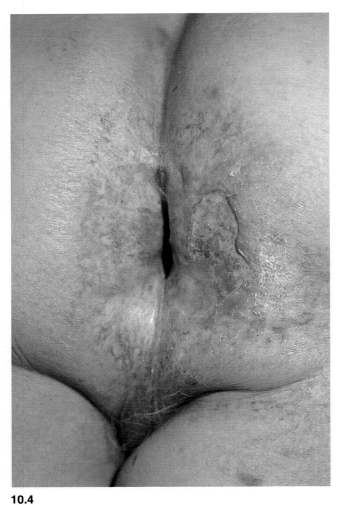

10.4
Chronic radiation dermatitis with an ulceration. The x-ray therapy had been given to treat pruritus ani.

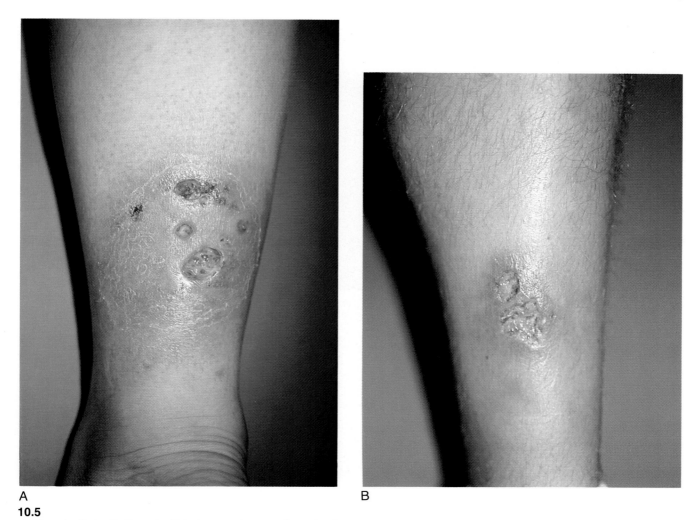

A

B

10.5

A, Panniculitis. *B*, Panniculitis in a patient with early rheumatoid arthritis.

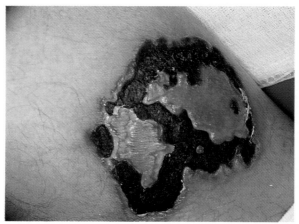

10.6

Factitial ulceration due to application of lye to the skin. Note the angulated borders.

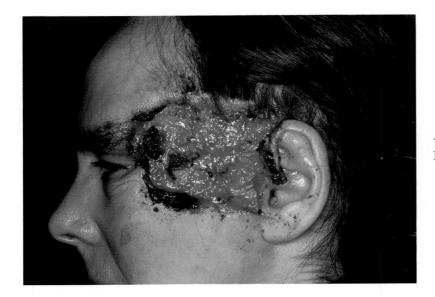

10.7
Long-neglected primary basal cell carcinoma.

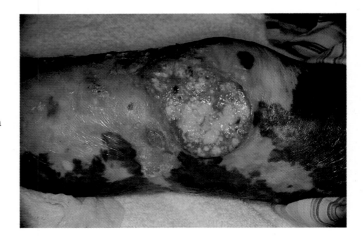

10.8
Squamous cell carcinoma in the scars associated with dystrophic epidermolysis bullosa.

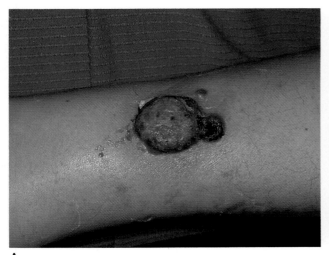

A

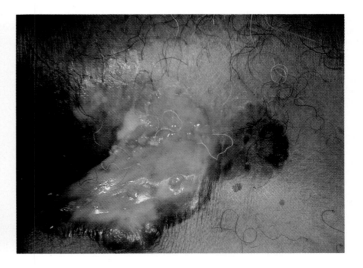

10.9
A, B, Ulcerating malignant melanoma.

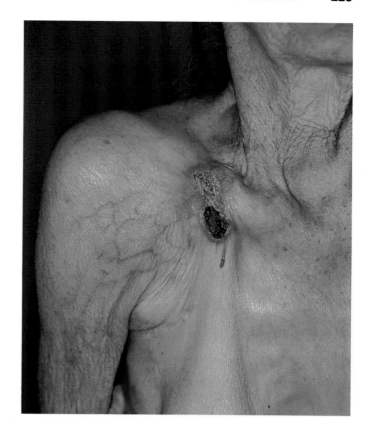

10.10
Metastatic breast carcinoma.

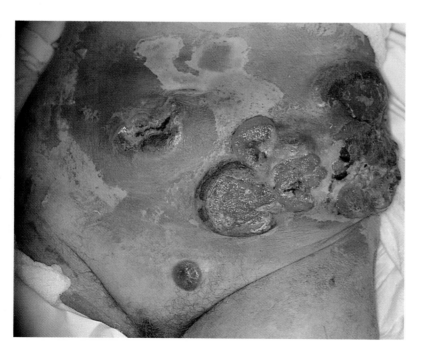

10.11
Tumors in advanced mycosis fungoides.

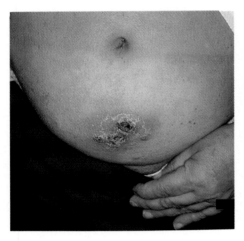

10.12
Cutaneous Hodgkin's disease.

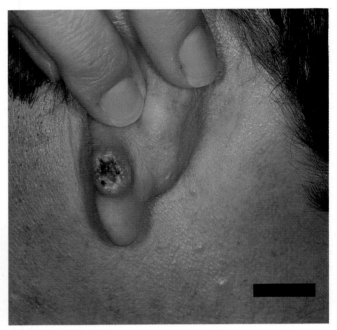

10.14
Keratoacanthoma.

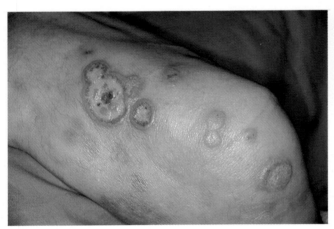

10.13
Lymphoma, large cell anaplastic variant (formerly known as reticulum cell sarcoma).[2]

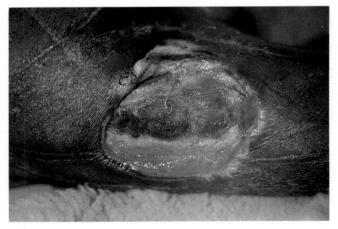

10.15
Decubitus ulceration. This lesion usually has an overhanging (undermined) border.

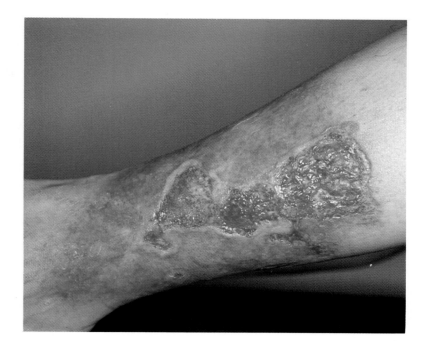

10.16
Pyoderma gangrenosum, classic presentation
in a patient with regional enteritis.

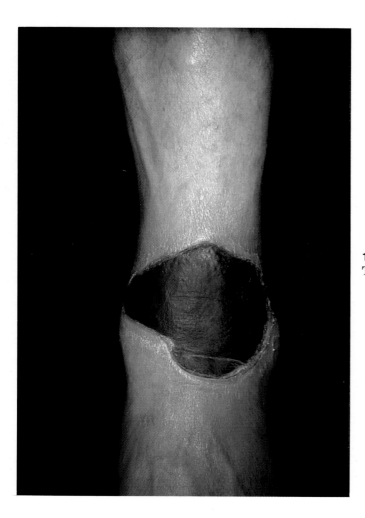

10.17
Traumatic ulceration.

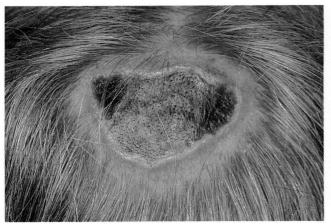

10.18
Pressure necrosis of the scalp after coronary artery bypass surgery with hypothermia.

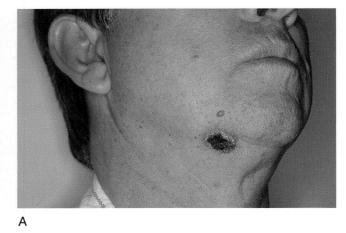

A

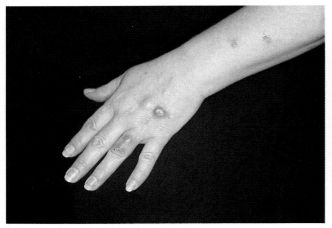

10.19
Atypical mycobacterial infection. Sporotrichoid spread of ulcerated nodules.

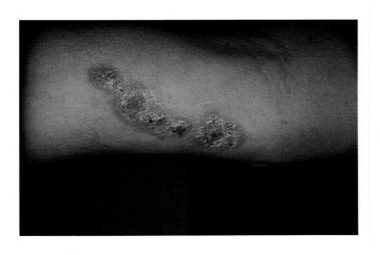

B
10.20
A, B, Blastomycosis.

10.21
Sporotrichosis.

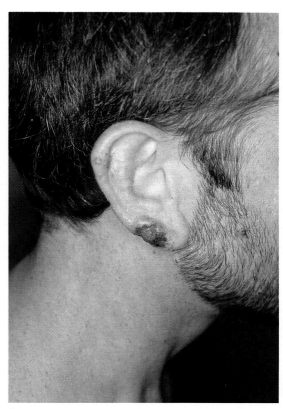

A

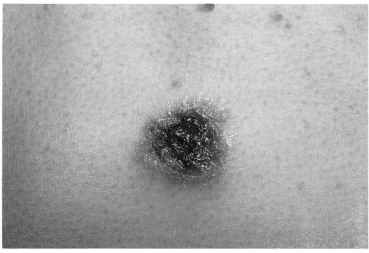

B

10.22
Cryptococcosis. *A,* In an HIV-positive man. *B,* In a patient on immunosuppressive therapy.

10.23
Erythema induratum, a chronic panniculitis.

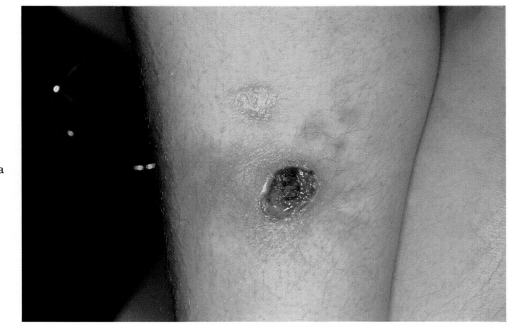

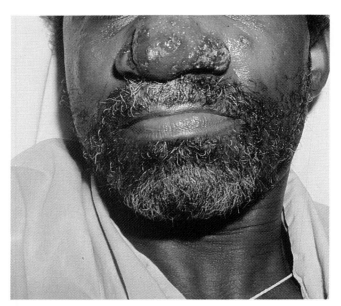

10.24
Leishmaniasis. Ulcerating nodules on the nose.[12]

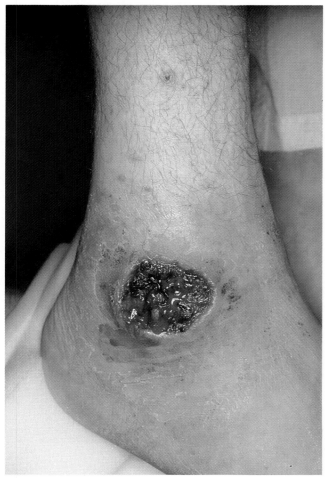

10.25
Wegener's granulomatosis.

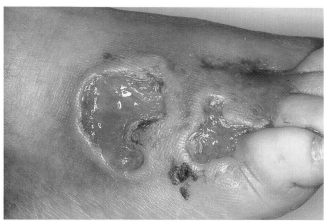

10.26
Rheumatoid vasculitis.

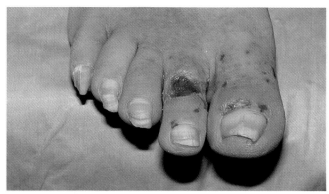

10.29
Atherosclerotic peripheral vascular disease.

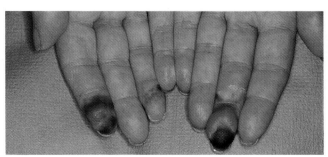

10.27
Polyarteritis nodosa due to hepatitis B antigenemia.[5]

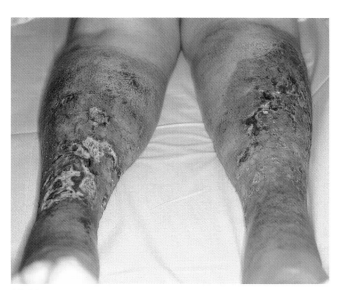

10.30
Ulcerating necrobiosis lipoidica diabeticorum.[3]

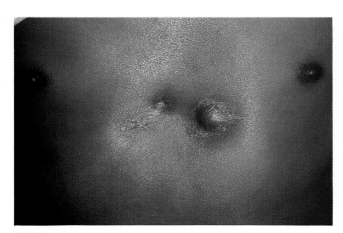

10.28
Actinomycosis. An ulcerating nodule.[12]

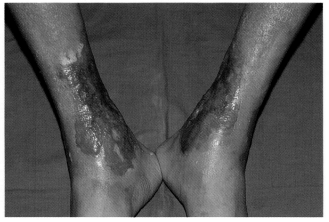

10.31
Stasis dermatitis with bilateral ulcerations over the medial malleoli.[5]

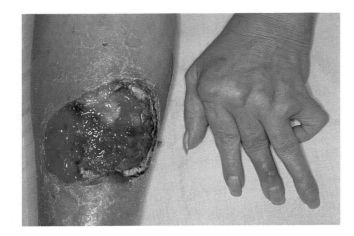

10.32
Pyoderma gangrenosum–like lesion in Felty's syndrome (rheumatoid arthritis with hypersplenism).

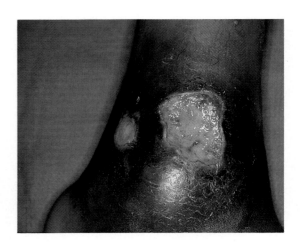

10.33
Sickle cell anemia.

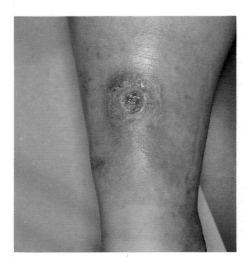

10.34
Antiphospholipid antibody syndrome.

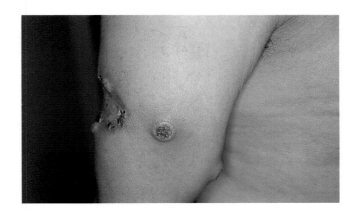

10.35
Halogenoderma.

GENITAL ULCERATIONS

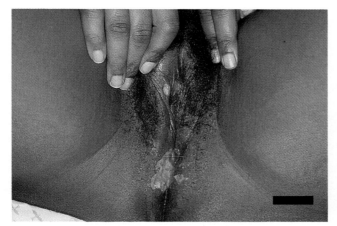

10.36
Vulvar pyoderma gangrenosum.

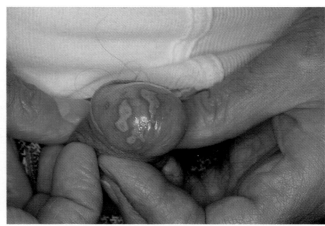

A

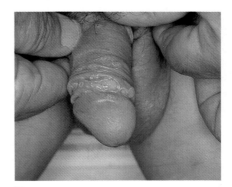

B

10.38
A, B, Chancroid.

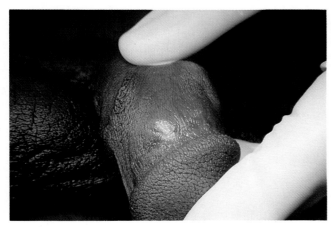

10.37
Chancre of primary syphilis.

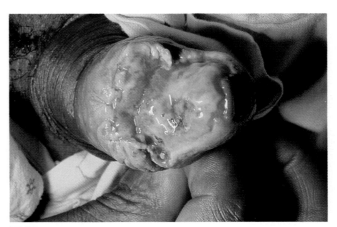

10.39
Granuloma inguinale.

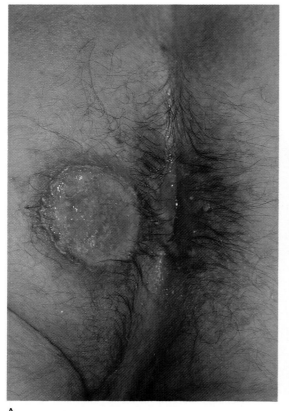

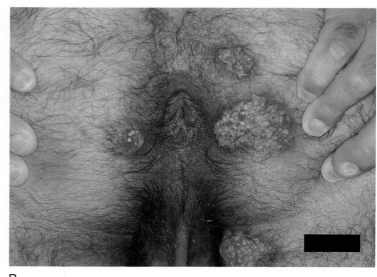

A   B

10.40
A, B, Herpes simplex infection in an HIV-positive man.[5]

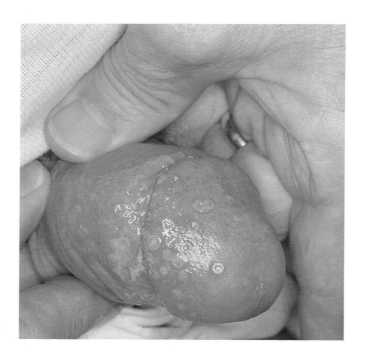

10.41
Primary herpes progenitalis.

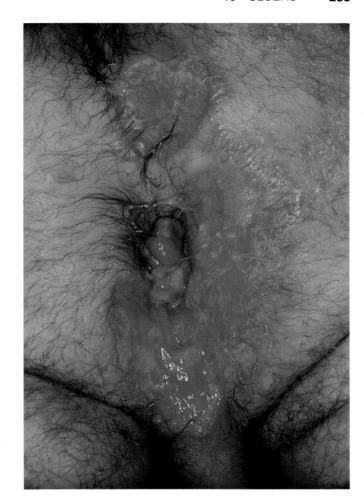

10.42
Tuberculosis of the perianal skin.

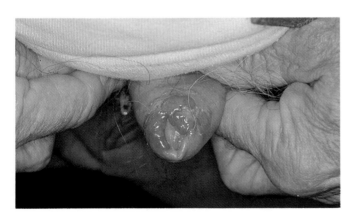

10.43
Erythroplasia of Queyrat. Squamous cell carcinoma on the penis.

URTICARIAL LESIONS

Urticaria is due to the accumulation of fluid within the upper dermis. The epidermis is stretched and the tightening results in the prominent follicular dilation commonly observed. Urticaria may also be erythematous because of the frequently dilated superficial blood vessels. Urticaria is a transient phenomenon that resolves with few, if any, residuals (Table IX). Histamine and/or other vasoactive amines and vasoactive substances are involved in many cases of urticaria.

TABLE IX
Urticaria: Classification and Differential Diagnosis

I. Acute and chronic urticaria
   Etiologies and provoking causes
   1. Drugs
   2. Foods and food additives
   3. Inhalants
   4. Infections
   5. Psychological factors
   6. General medical disorders (lymphoproliferative disorders, endocrinopathies, pregnancy)
II. Contact urticaria
   Etiologies and provoking causes
   1. Foods and food additives
   2. Drugs
   3. Animal saliva or dander
   4. Grass pollen
   5. Caterpillars
   6. Algae and lichens
   7. Industrial exposure
      a. Ammonium persulfate
      b. Platinum
III. Immune complex urticaria, urticarial vasculitis
   Etiologies and associated conditions
   1. Systemic lupus erythematosus
   2. Hepatitis B
IV. Physical urticaria
   Types of physical urticaria and related disorders
   1. Dermatographism
   2. Pressure urticaria
   3. Solar urticaria (various types)
   4. Cold urticaria
      a. Familial cold urticaria
      b. Idiopathic cold urticaria
      c. Cold urticaria caused by cryoglobulins, cold agglutinins
      d. Cold erythema
      e. Cold reflex urticaria
   5. Heat urticaria (localized)
   6. Cholinergic urticaria or pruritus
   7. Aquagenic urticaria or pruritus
   8. Vibratory angioedema
V. Angioedema
   1. Hereditary angioedema

Adapted from Rook A: Textbook of Dermatology. 4th ed. Blackwell Scientific Publications, Oxford, 1986.

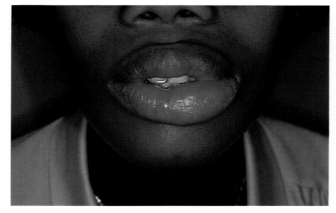

11.1
Angioedema. Urticaria of the mucous membrane; a deeper swelling is sometimes noted.

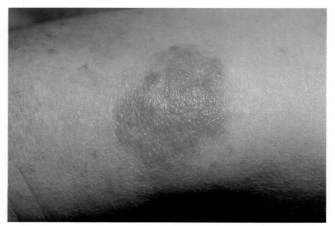

11.2
Wells' syndrome (eosinophilic cellulitis).

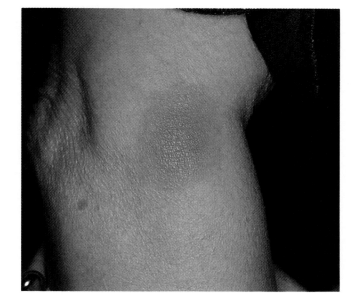

11.3
Fixed drug eruption. An early lesion may be manifested as an urticarial plaque. This lesion frequently resolves with macular hyperpigmentation. The cause in this patient was a phenolphthalein-containing laxative.

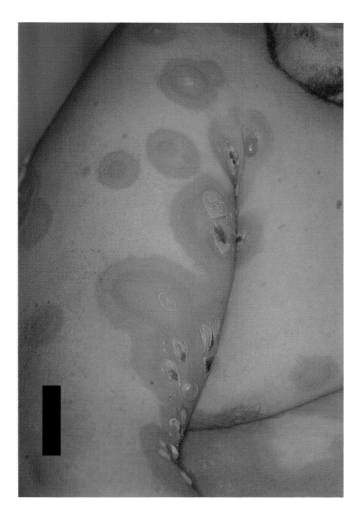

11.4
Bullous pemphigoid. Urticarial plaques with bullae and erosions. On rare occasions the urticarial lesions may be the only manifestation of this immunobullous disease.

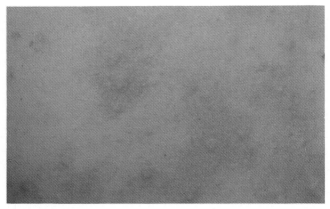

11.5
Cholinergic urticaria. These patients have small urticarial lesions that may be precipitated by exercise, heat, or emotional stress.[5]

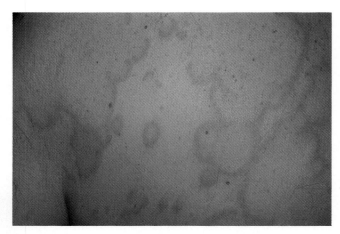

11.7
Polycyclic lesions of urticaria.

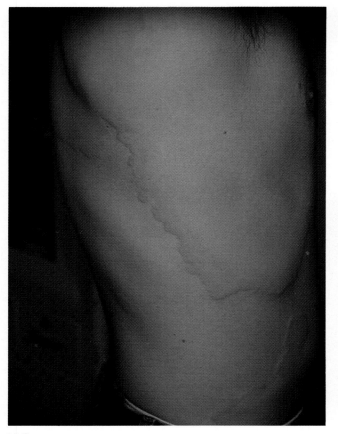

11.6
Giant urticarial lesion of urticaria.

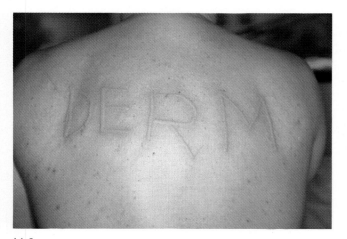

11.8
Dermatographism is more common in patients with urticaria, but it occurs in about 5% of the normal population.

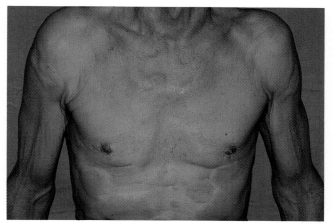

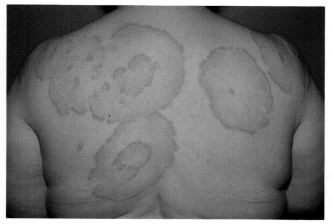

11.9
Urticarial vasculitis. This patient's urticarial lesions are histopathologically leukocytoclastic vasculitis. Clinically the lesions are different from nonvasculitic urticaria in that they are less pruritic, last longer (more than 4 to 5 hours and often more than 24 hours), and frequently resolve with a bruise.[5]

11.11
Figurate erythema.[4]

11.12
Erythema toxicum in a newborn. A transient phenomenon.

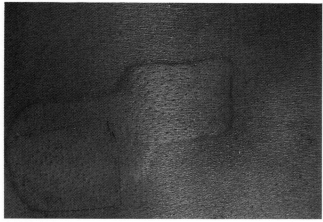

11.10
Cold urticaria. An ice cube was placed on the skin of this patient, inducing an urticarial lesion.[12]

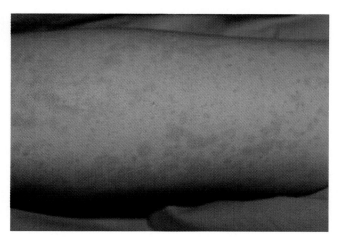

11.13
Juvenile rheumatoid arthritis with transient urticarial lesions.

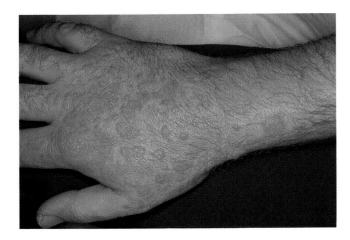

11.14
Erythema multiforme triggered by a recurrent herpes simplex virus infection.

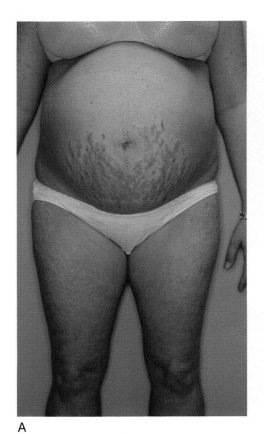

A

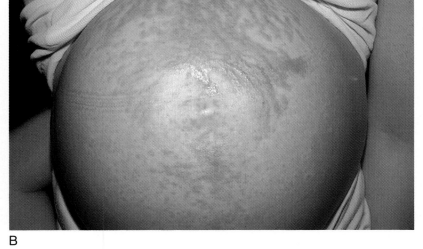

B

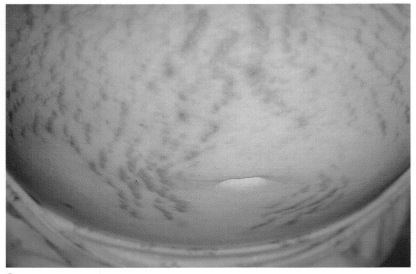

C

11.15
A to *C,* Pruritic urticarial papules and plaques of pregnancy.

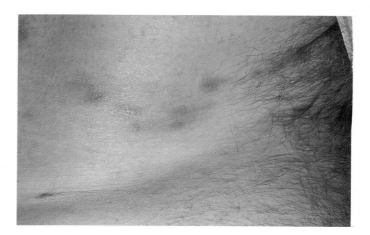

11.16
Scabies occasionally causes urticarial plaques.

ATROPHIC AND/OR SCLEROTIC LESIONS

Atrophy refers to a loss of tissue substance. Cutaneous atrophy can be epidermal, dermal, subcutaneous, or a combination of any of these layers. *Sclerosis* is a process in which excessive collagen is present.

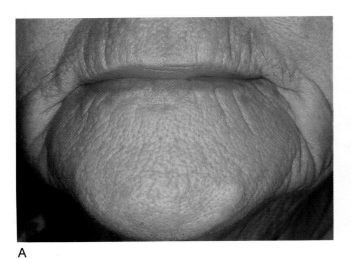

A

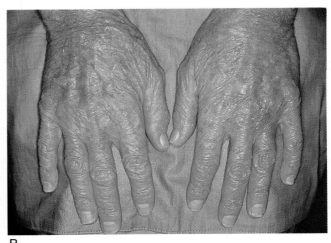

B

12.1

A, Actinic (solar) damage with elastosis. Aging of the skin results in changes that are more pronounced on exposed surfaces.[14] *B,* Actinic damage.[2]

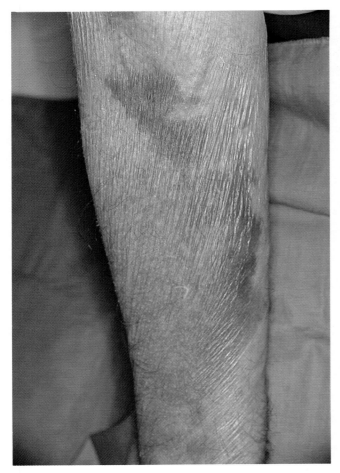

12.2
Corticosteroid-induced atrophy. This patient also has ecchymoses, which are another complication of corticosteroid therapy.[2]

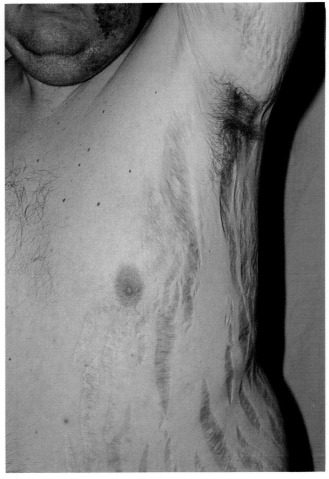

12.3
Corticosteroid-induced striae. This change combines epidermal and dermal atrophy.

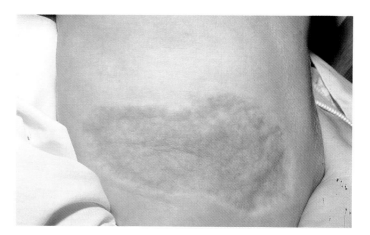

12.4
Localized idiopathic lipoatrophy.

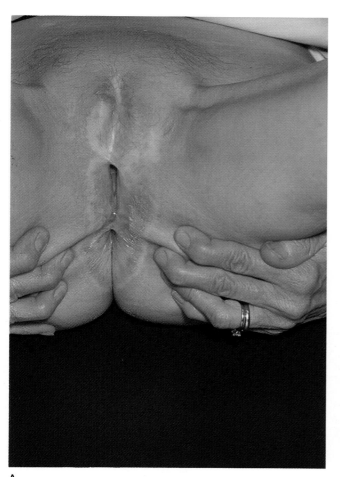

A

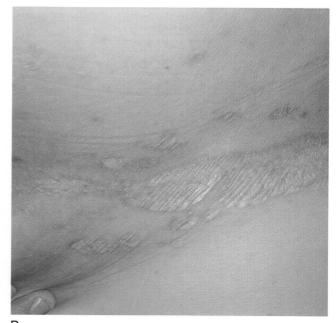

B

12.5
A, B, Lichen sclerosus et atrophicus.

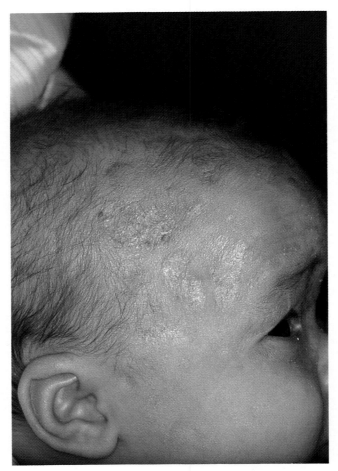

12.6
Neonatal lupus erythematosus.

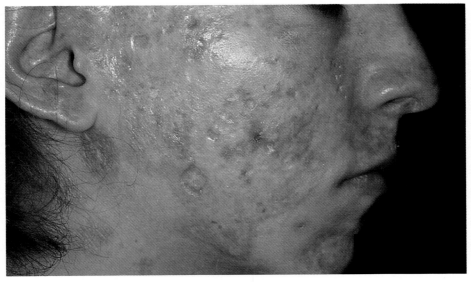

12.7
Discoid lupus erythematosus. Epidermal atrophy with scarring.

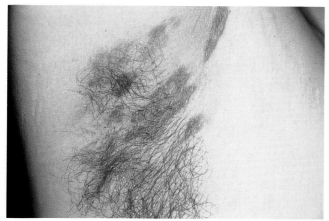

12.8
Atrophic (and inverse) lichen planus.

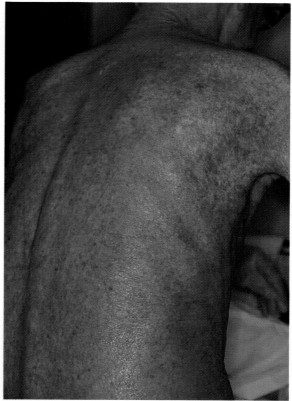

12.11
Sézary syndrome. A variant of mycosis fungoides or cutaneous T-cell lymphoma in which the patient has erythroderma with circulating T lymphocytes (Sézary cells).

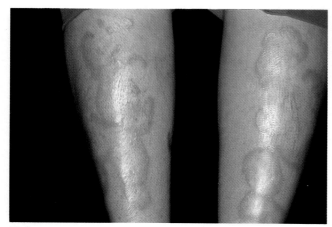

12.9
Necrobiosis lipoidica diabeticorum.

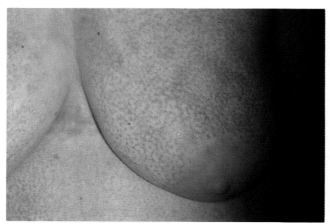

12.10
Poikiloderma atrophicans vasculare.

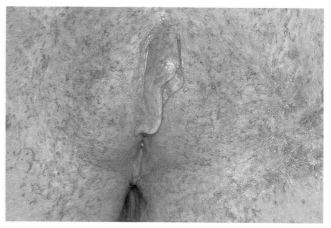

12.12
Radiation dermatitis.

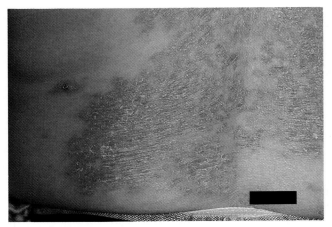

12.13
Poikilodermatous changes of chronic cutaneous lupus erythematosus.

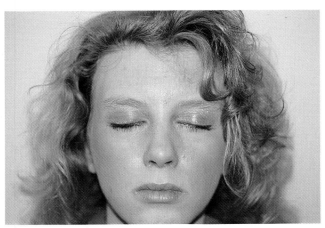

12.15
Heliotrope rash seen in dermatomyositis.

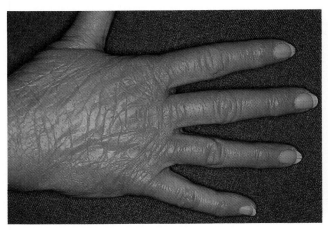

12.14
Poikiloderma of dermatomyositis.

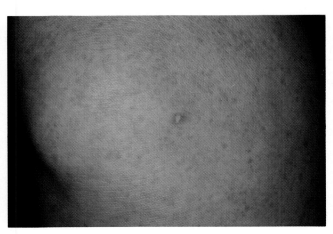

12.16
Degos' disease (malignant atrophic papulosis).

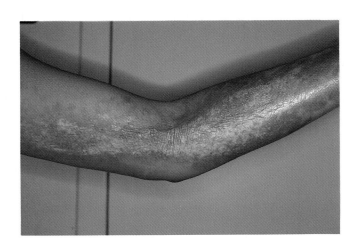

12.17
Linear scleroderma. There is epidermal atrophy in this dermal sclerotic disease.

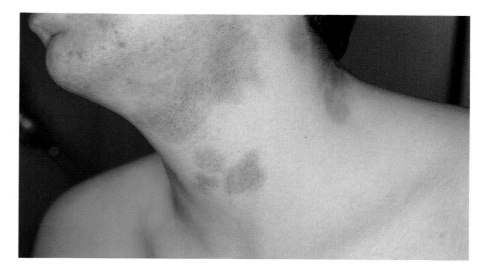

12.18
Lichen sclerosus et atrophicus and morphea (localized scleroderma) overlap.

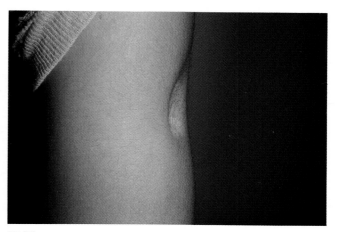

12.20
Corticosteroid-induced atrophy. This patient has a panatrophy of the skin after leakage of drug back into the skin after "intramuscular" injection of triamcinolone acetonide for the treatment of acute contact dermatitis.

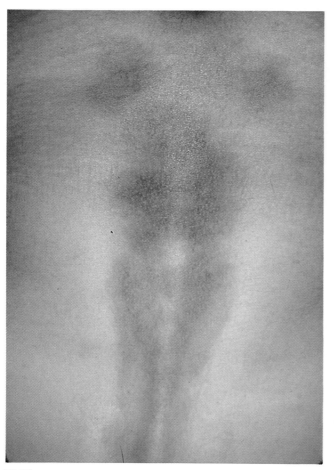

12.19
Atrophoderma of Pasini and Pierini. An idiopathic condition with dermal atrophy and occasionally epidermal atrophy. Perhaps it represents the end stage of morphea (localized scleroderma).

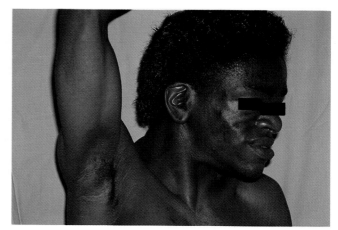

12.21
Partial lipodystrophy with acanthosis nigricans.

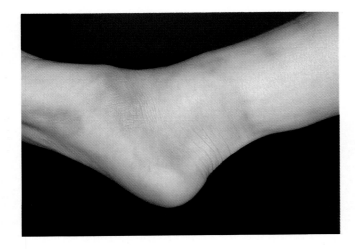

12.22
Lipoatrophy after panniculitis.

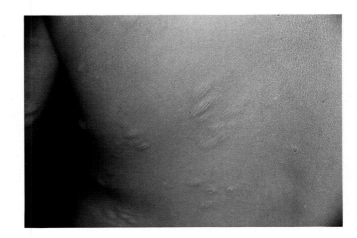

12.23
Anetoderma after secondary syphilis. This change is due to loss of elastic fibers, which results in a softened out-pouching of the skin.[10]

SCLEROSIS

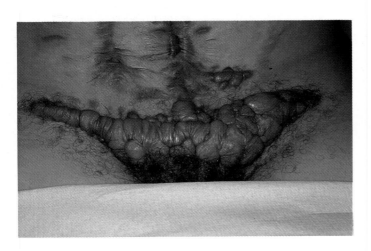

12.24
Keloids.

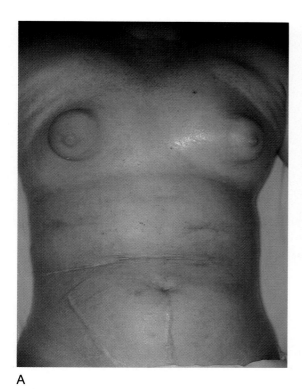

A

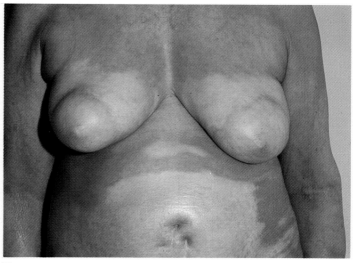

B

12.25
A, B, Generalized morphea. A rare sclerodermatous condition in which only the skin is involved, but the involvement is diffuse. The nipples on this woman are the only uninvolved area and thus they protrude.

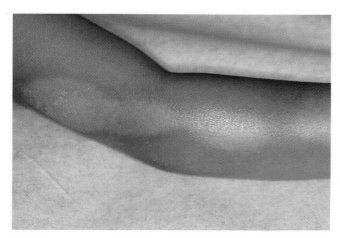

12.26
Linear scleroderma.

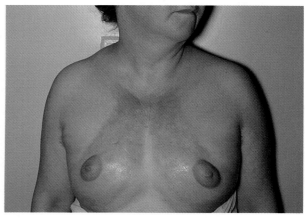

12.27
Morphea.

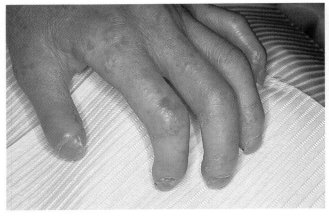

12.28
Progressive systemic sclerosis with sclerodactyly.

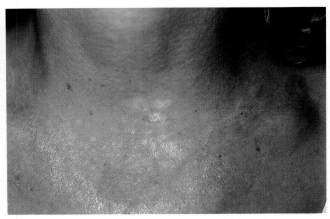

12.31
Sclerodermoid changes in porphyria cutanea tarda.

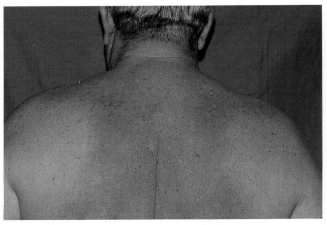

12.29
Scleredema adultorum of Buschke. A hardening of the skin on the upper trunk due to infiltration of mucinous material. This occurs primarily in men who are diabetics.[5]

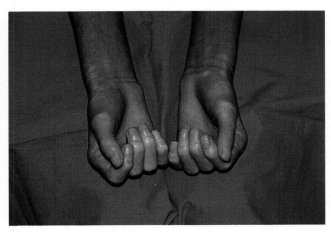

12.32
Scleromyxedema.

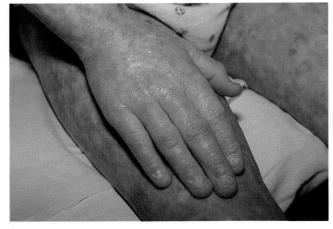

12.30
Chronic graft-versus-host disease. In its chronic form, it often simulates scleroderma.

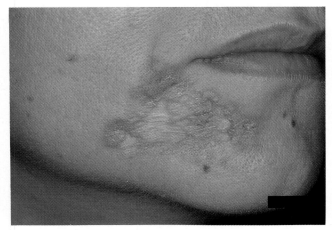

12.33
Scarring of chronic cutaneous (discoid) lupus erythematosus.

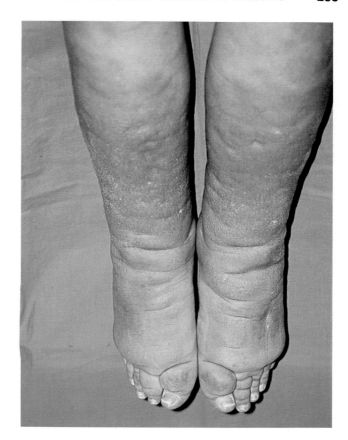

12.34
Pretibial myxedema.

CONFIGURATIONS

13

ANNULAR LESIONS

An annular configuration is one in which the border is active, either with elevation of a dermal infiltrate or with scale.

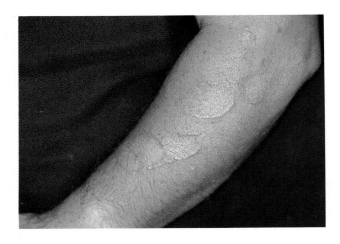

13.1
Granuloma annulare.

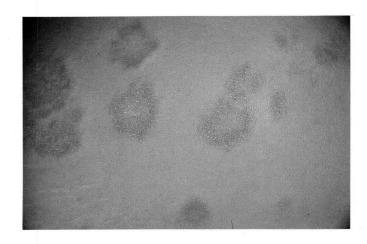

13.2
Sarcoidosis.

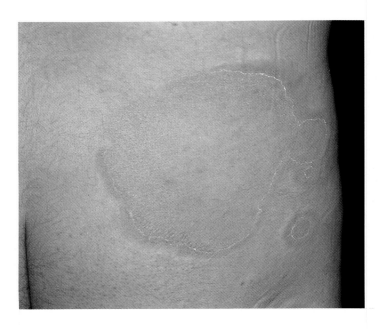

13.3
Erythema annulare centrifugum.

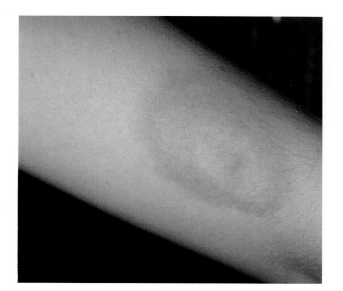

13.4
Erythema chronicum migrans of Lyme disease.

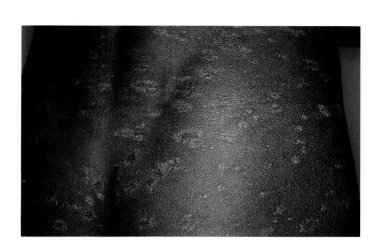

13.5
Secondary syphilis.

13.6
Lichen planus.

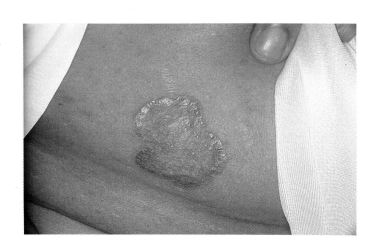
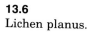

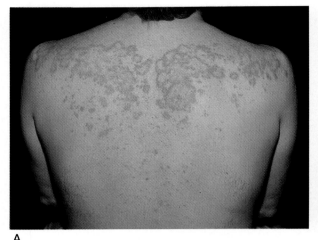

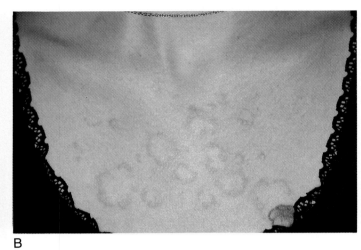

A

B

13.7

A, B, Subacute cutaneous lupus erythematosus.

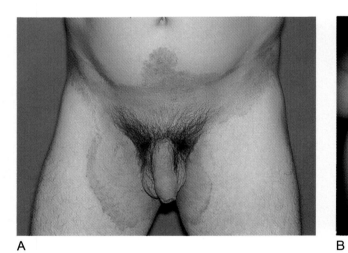

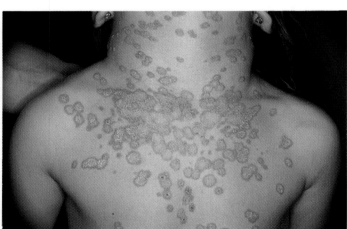

A

B

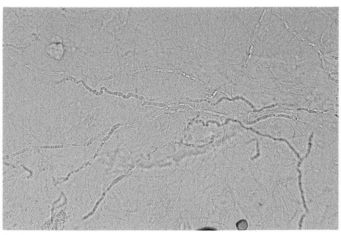

C

13.8

A, Tinea cruris. *B,* Tinea corporis. *C,* Potassium hydroxide examination in a patient with a superficial fungal infection of the skin, such as those pictured in *A* and *B.*

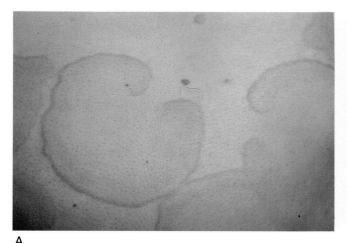

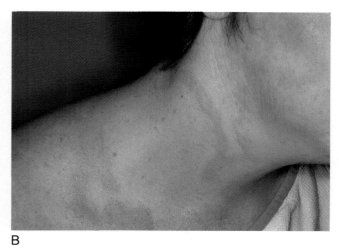

A

B

13.9

A, B, Urticaria.

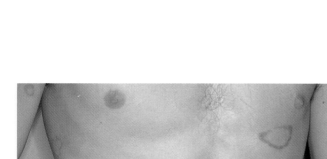

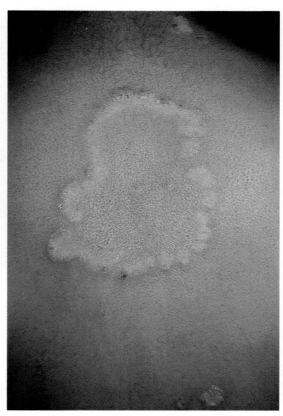

A

13.10

A, B, Psoriasis.

B

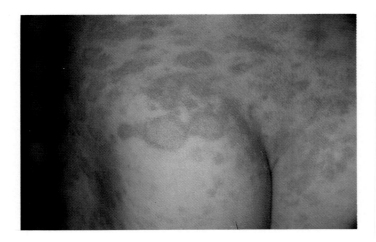

13.11
Purpura annularis telangiectoides.

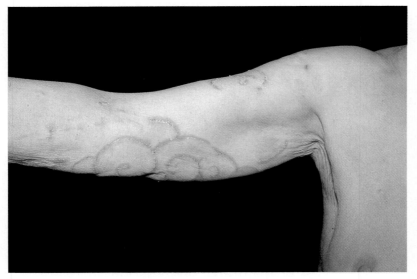

A
13.12
A, B, Mycosis fungoides (*A*[17]).

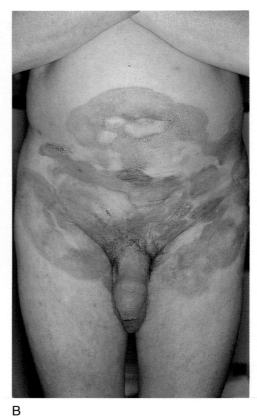

B

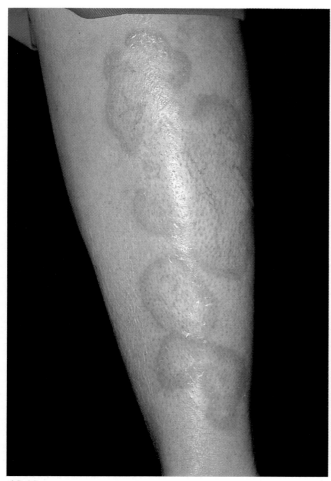

13.13
Necrobiosis lipoidica diabeticorum.

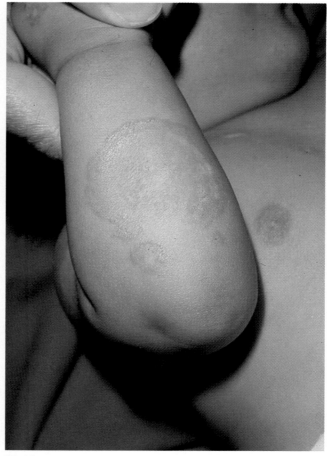

13.14
Neonatal lupus erythematosus.

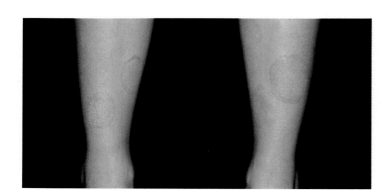

13.15
Nummular eczema.

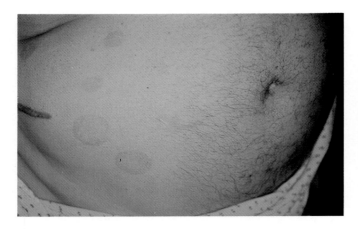

13.16
Pityriasis rotunda. Rare, round hyperpigmented patches, most common in dark-skinned individuals. This condition may be associated with nutritional disease or hepatocellular carcinoma.[7]

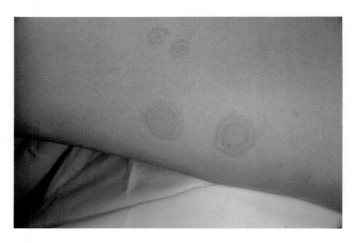

13.17
Erythema multiforme.

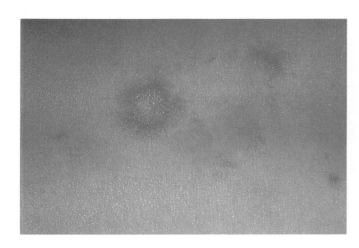

13.18
Benign lymphocytic infiltrate.

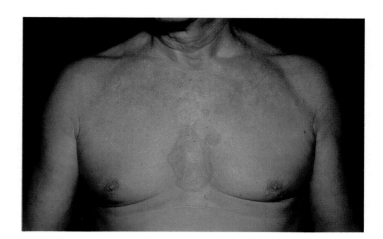

13.19
Annular seborrheic dermatitis.[5]

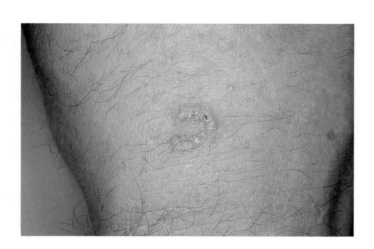

13.20
Actinic granuloma.[3]

LINEAR LESIONS

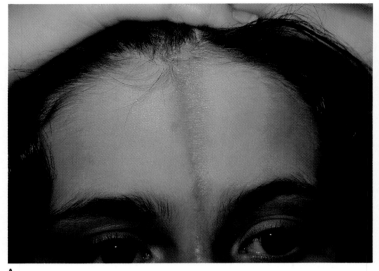

A

14.1
A, B, Linear scleroderma, en coup de sabre.

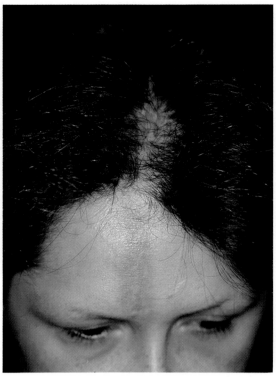

B

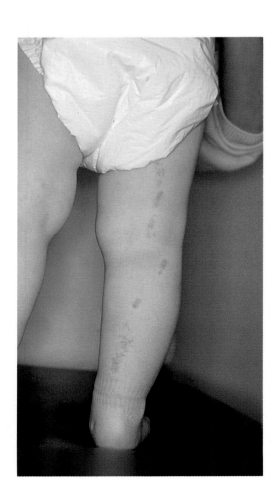

14.2
Lichen striatus.

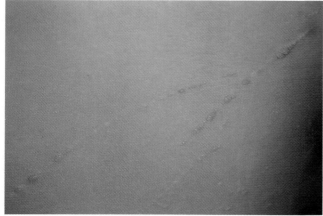

A

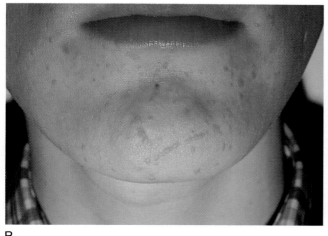

B

14.3
A, B, Warts. These lesions were inoculated after trauma to the skin.

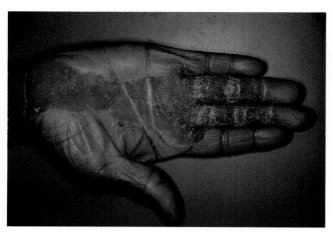

14.4
Linear epidermal nevus.

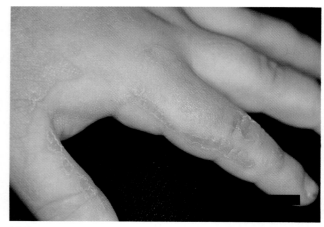

14.5
Linear porokeratosis.

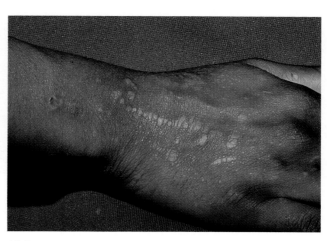

14.6
Linear lichen planus due to Koebner's phenomenon.

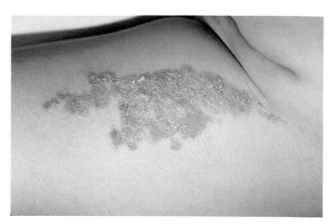

14.7
Inflammatory linear verrucous epidermal nevus.

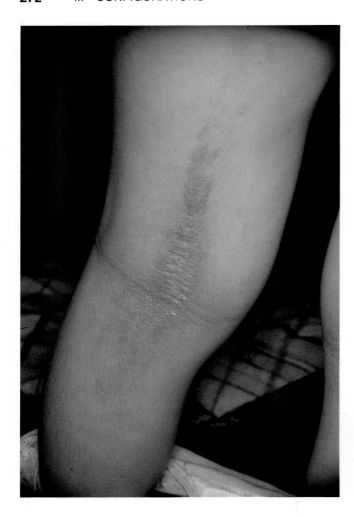

14.8
Ichthyosis hystrix. This may be a process identical to inflammatory linear verrucous epidermal nevus.

14.9
Nevus sebaceus of Jadassohn.

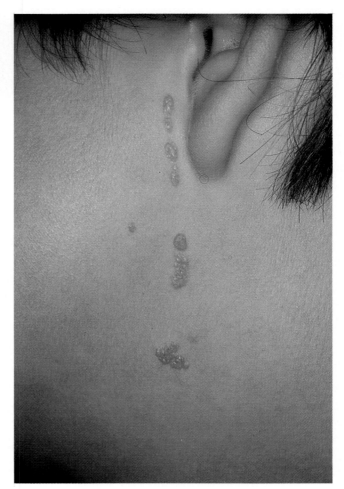

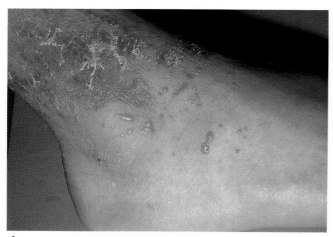

A

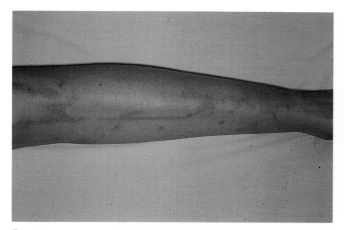

B
14.10
A, B, Contact dermatitis.

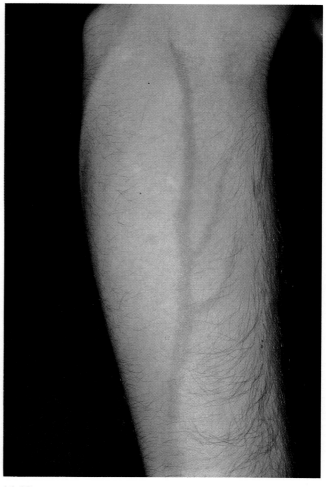

14.12
Superficial phlebitis after nitrogen mustard intravenous therapy.[6]

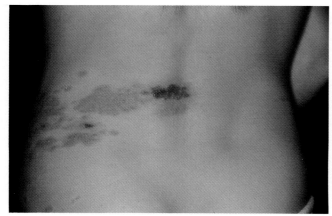

14.11
Herpes zoster.

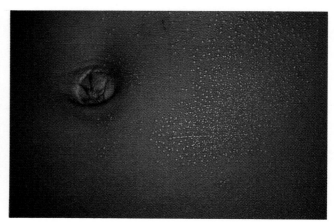

14.13
Lichen nitidus.[2]

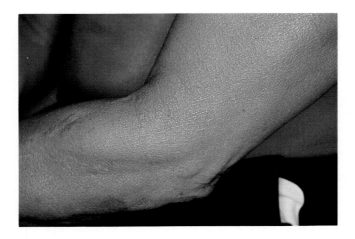

14.14
Lichen myxedematosus (papular mucinosis).

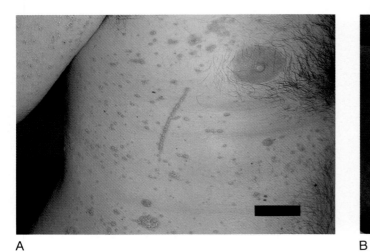

A

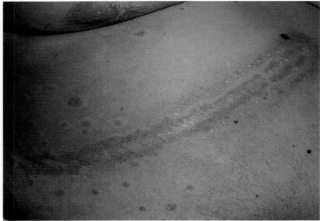

B

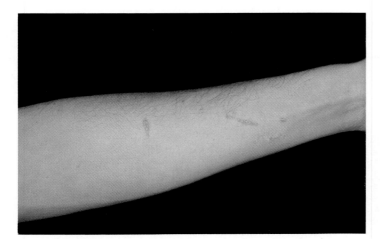

C

14.15
A to *C,* Psoriasis. Koebner's phenomenon.

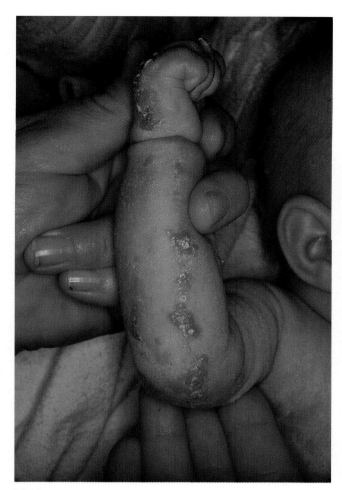

14.16
Incontinentia pigmenti.

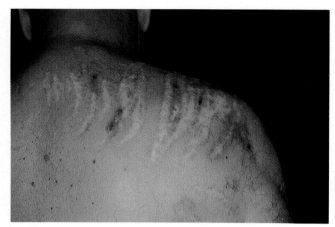

14.18
Neurodermatitis. Linear scars from deep excoriation.

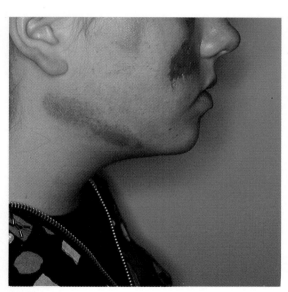

14.19
Factitial dermatitis.

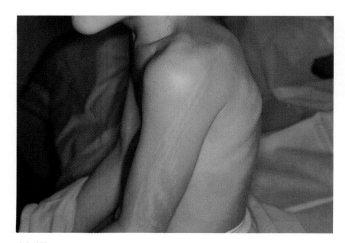

14.17
Hypomelanosis of Ito (incontinentia pigmenti achromians)

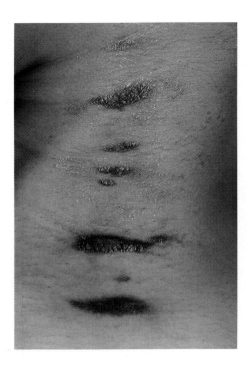

14.20
Sarcoidosis.[8]

SPOROTRICHOID LESIONS

Linearity is present, but these lesions are usually nodules with normal skin spaced between the lesions.

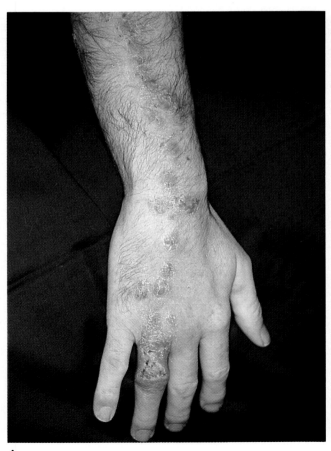

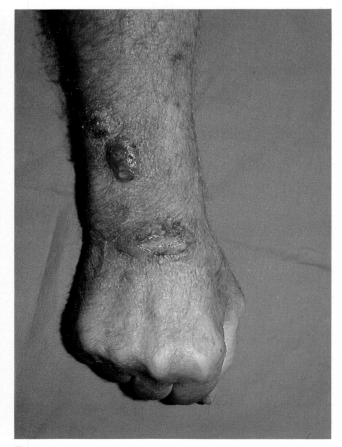

A

B

14.21
A, B, Sporotrichosis (*A*[6]).

14.22
Atypical mycobacterial infection (*Mycobacterium marinum*).

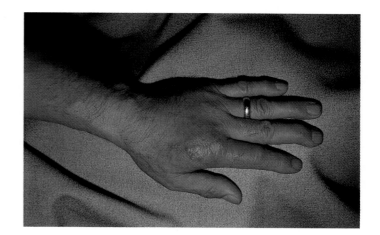

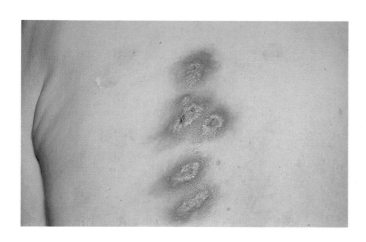

14.23
Leishmaniasis.[17]

GYRATE OR SERPIGINOUS LESIONS

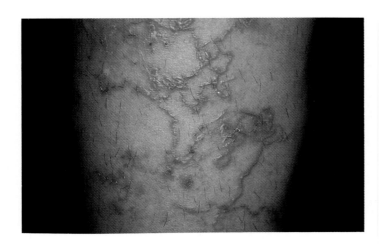

15.1
Cutaneous larva migrans.[3]

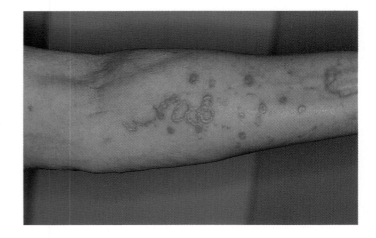

15.2
Granuloma annulare.

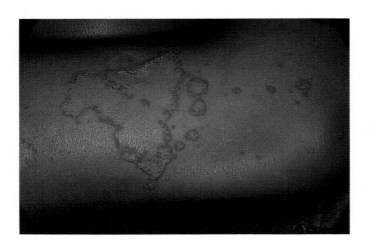

15.3
Porokeratosis of Mibelli.[3]

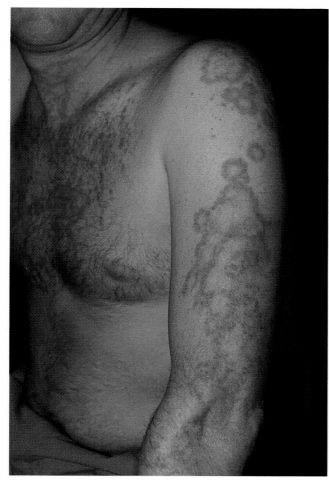

15.4
Subacute cutaneous lupus erythematosus.

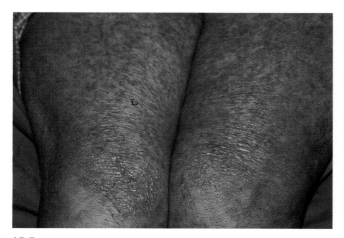

15.5
Parapsoriasis variegata.

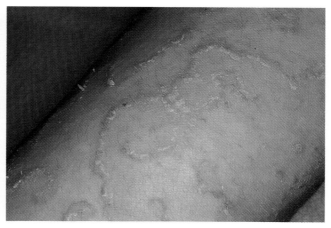

15.6
Erythrokeratodermia variabilis. An autosomal dominant disorder that affects only the skin.[3]

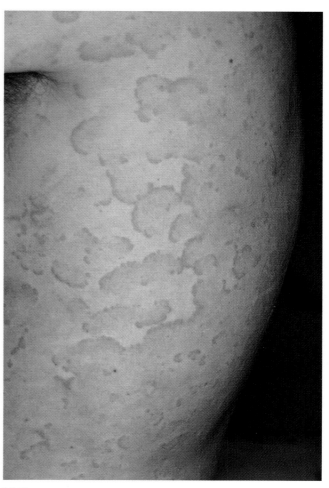

15.7
Erythema annulare centrifugum.

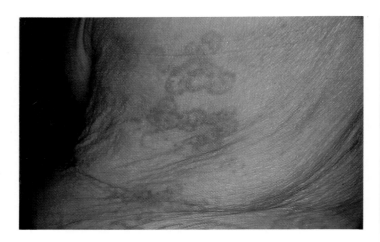

15.8
Erythema gyratum repens.

15.9
Elastosis perforans serpiginosa.

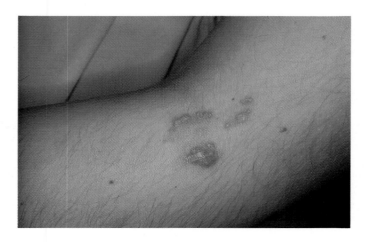

GROUPED OR HERPETIFORM LESIONS

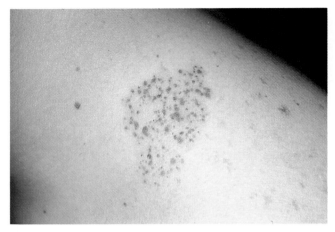

16.1
Nevus spilus.

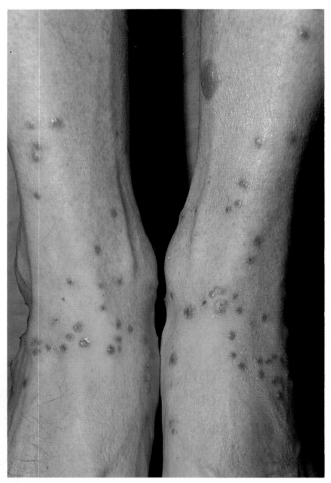

16.3
Insect bites are often grouped. In this case, fleas were the cause.

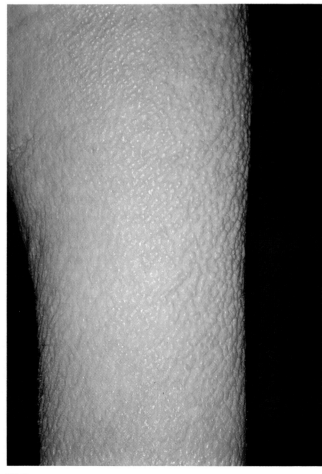

16.2
Papular mucinosis.

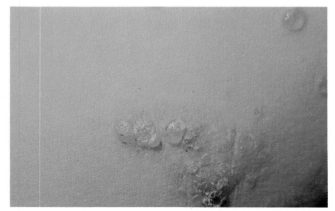

16.4
Lymphangioma circumscriptum.

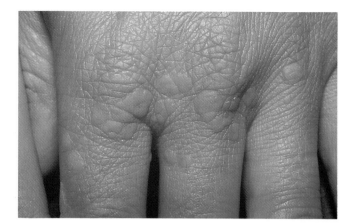

16.5
Epidermodysplasia verruciformis. An autosomal recessive disorder in which there is a defect in immunity to infection with human papillomavirus, particularly Types 5 and 8. In addition, these patients may develop multiple squamous cell carcinomas.

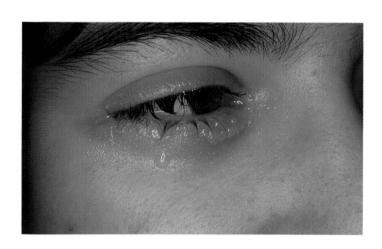

16.6
Herpes simplex.

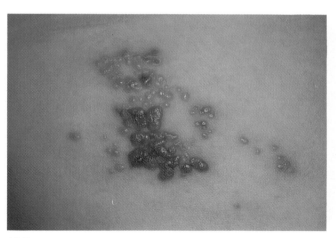

16.7
Herpes zoster.[6]

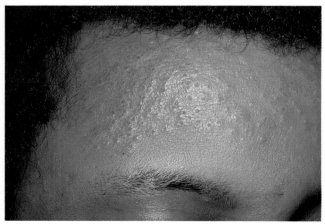

16.8
Eczema herpeticum (herpes simplex infection).

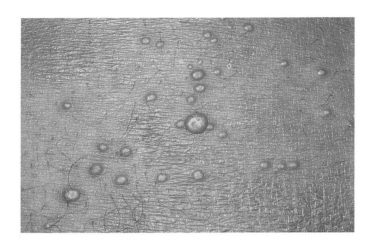

16.9
Multiple molluscum contagiosum.

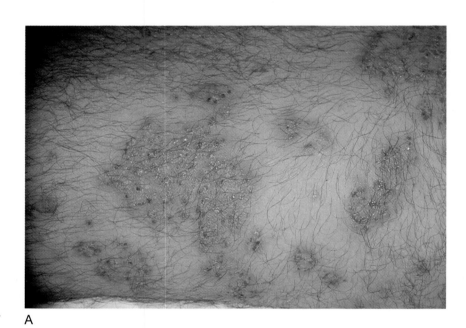

A

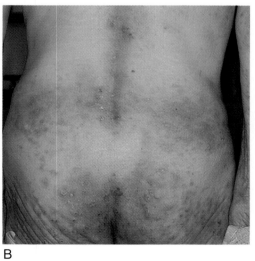

B

16.10
A, B, Dermatitis herpetiformis.

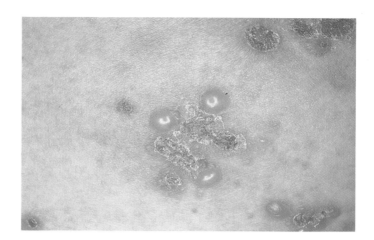

16.11
Vesicular pemphigoid.

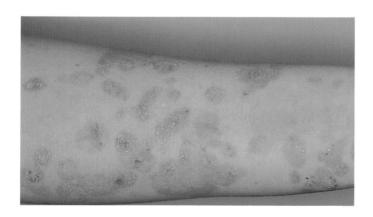

16.12
Herpes gestationis.

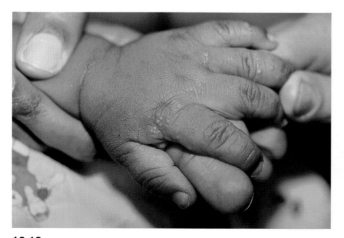

16.13
Acropustulosis of infancy.

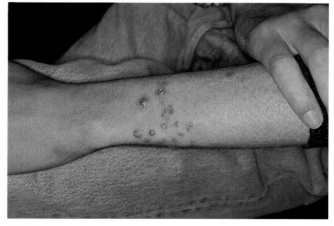

16.14
Fungal granuloma in an HIV-infected patient.

RETICULATED OR NETLIKE LESIONS

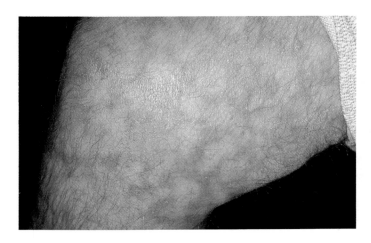

17.1
Erythema ab igne.

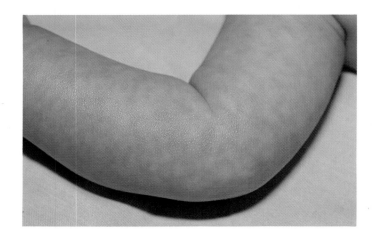

17.2
Cutis marmorata.

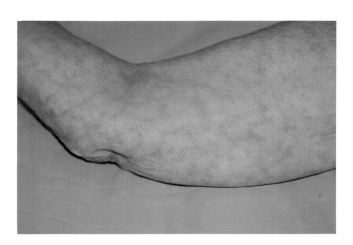

17.3
Livedo reticularis. A reaction pattern in which the lesions have a dusky to purpuric, netlike appearance. This pattern is suggestive of several disorders (Table X).

TABLE X
Differential Diagnosis of Livedo Reticularis

Congenital
    Cutis marmorata telangiectatica congenita
    Rothmund-Thomson syndrome
Physiologic
    Cutis marmorata
Blood vessel disease
    Arteriosclerosis
    Arteritis
    Leukocytoclastic vasculitis
    Cutaneous polyarteritis nodosa
    Lupus erythematosus
    Dermatomyositis
    Rheumatoid arthritis
    Pancreatitis
Intravascular obstruction
    Emboli
    Anticardiolipin syndrome
    Cryoglobulinemia, cryofibrinogenemia
    Oxalosis
    Thrombocythemia, polycythemia
Pharmacologic
    Amantidine
    Catecholamines
Idiopathic
    Livedoid vasculitis

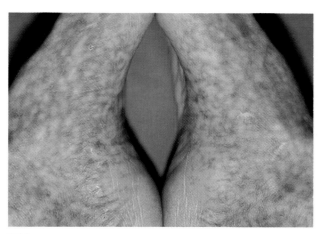

17.4
Livedoid vasculitis or atrophie blanche.

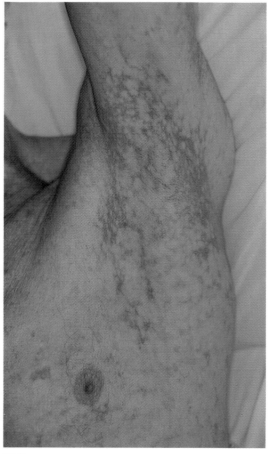

17.5
Dyskeratosis congenita.

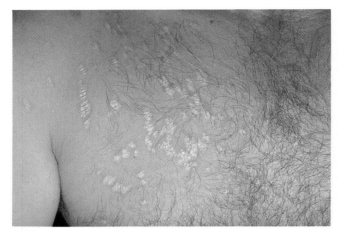

17.6
Lichen sclerosus et atrophicus.

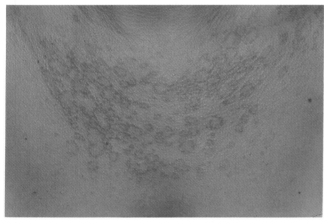

17.7
Reticular erythematous mucinosis.

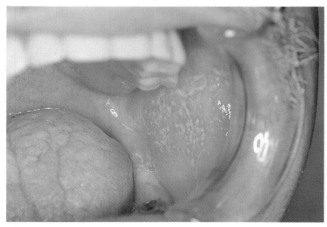

17.8
Lichen planus.

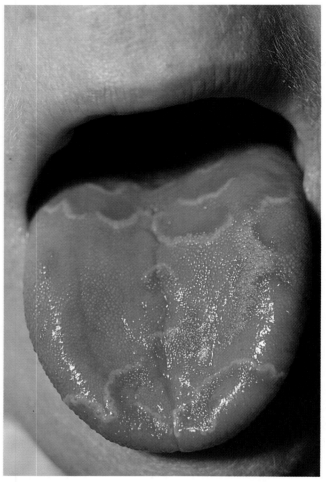

17.9
Geographic tongue.

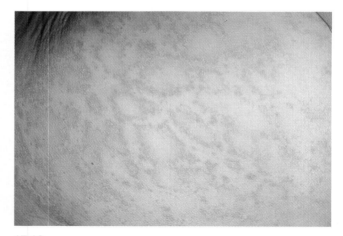

17.10
Parakeratosis variegata (retiform parapsoriasis). A form of large plaque parapsoriasis.

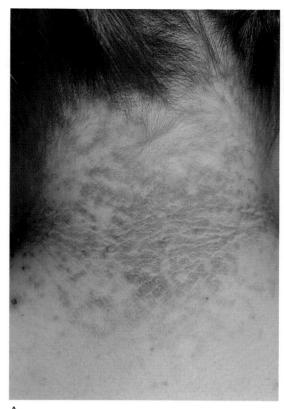

A

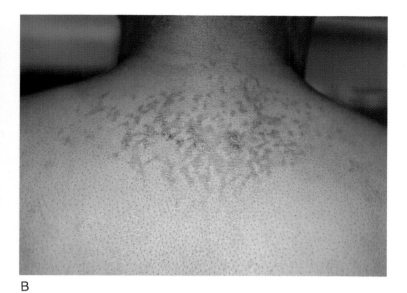

B

17.11
A, B, Confluent and reticulated papillomatosis.

17.12
Fifth disease.[6]

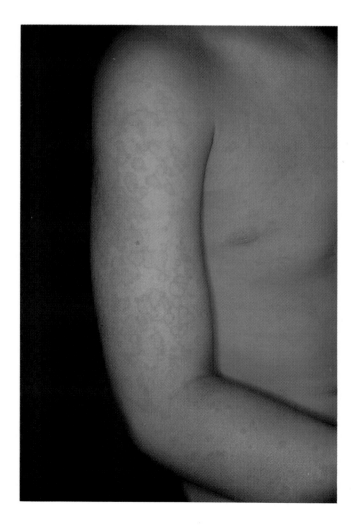

DISTRIBUTIONS AND REGIONAL PREDILECTIONS

GENERALIZED DISORDERS

These disorders traditionally occur on all body surfaces. There may be a certain predilection for a specific area (e.g., vitiligo tends to be periorificial, and psoriasis favors extensor surfaces such as the elbows and knees), but in many patients the disease is widespread. This is in contrast to conditions described in subsequent sections in which there is a disease limited to, or more prominent on, the palms and soles, sun-exposed surfaces, intertriginous surfaces, mucous membranes, scalp, or nails.

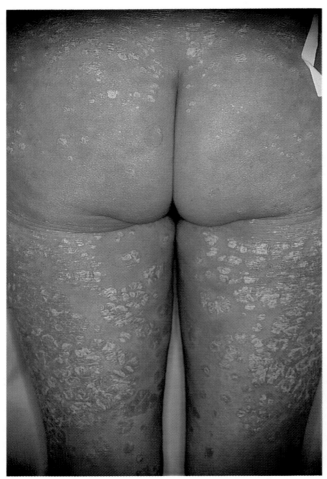

18.1
Psoriasis vulgaris.

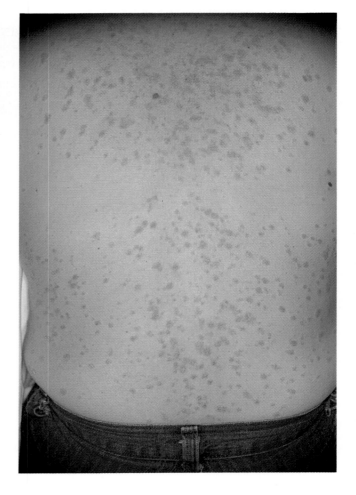

18.2
Guttate psoriasis.

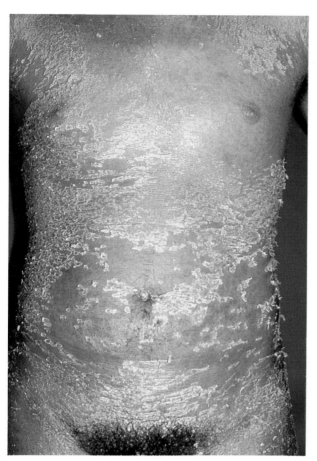

18.3
Psoriatic erythroderma.

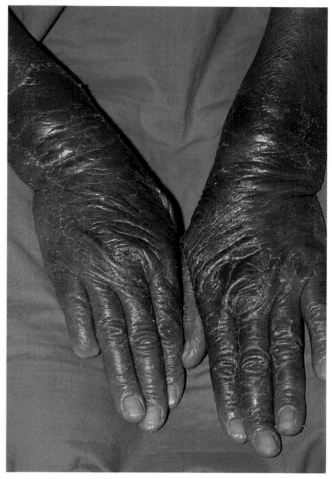

18.5
Erythroderma, drug-induced.[5]

18.4
Mycosis fungoides.

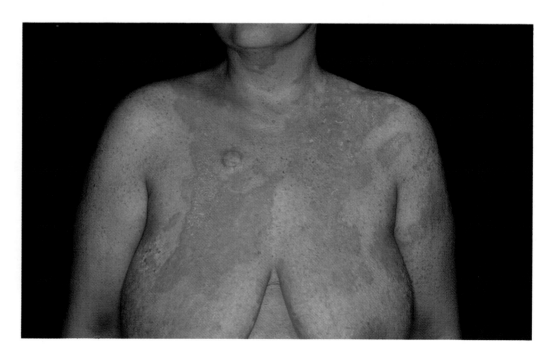

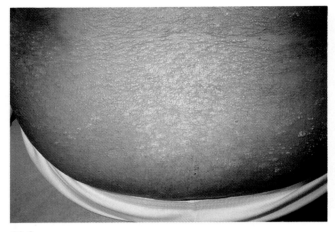

18.6
Generalized lichen planus.

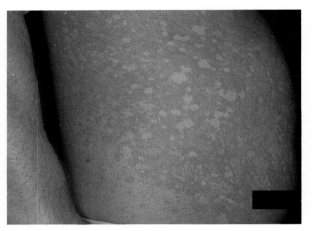

18.8
Pityriasis rubra pilaris.

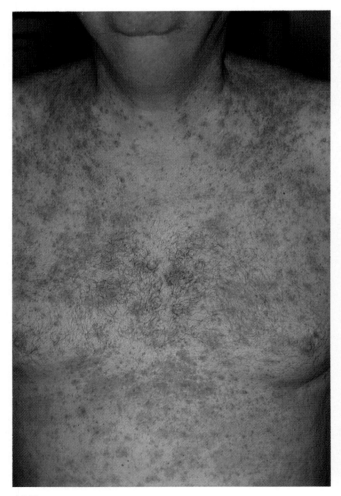

18.7
Drug eruption.

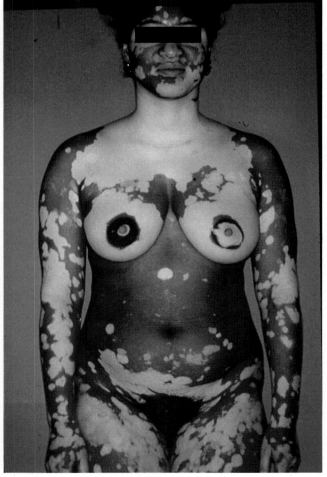

18.9
Vitiligo.

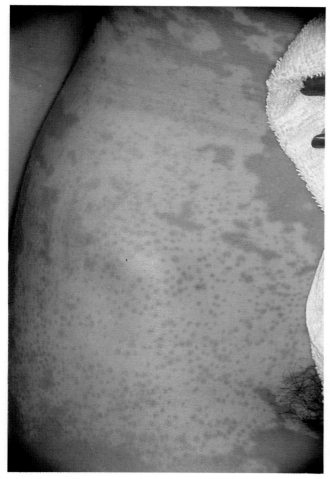

18.10
Vitiligo with repigmentation from psoralen plus ultraviolet A (PUVA) therapy.

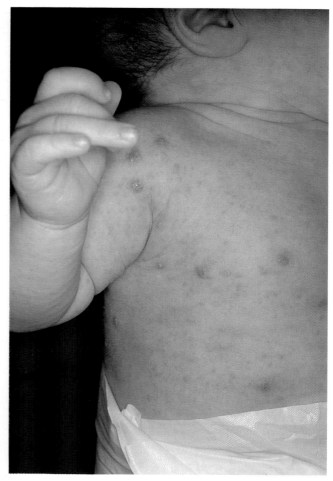

18.12
Scabies.

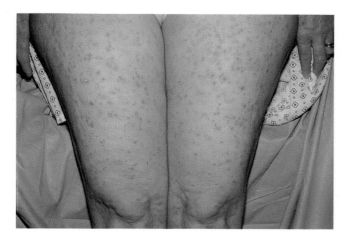

18.11
Pityriasis lichenoides et varioliformis acuta.

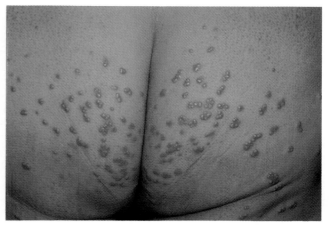

18.13
Eruptive xanthomas.

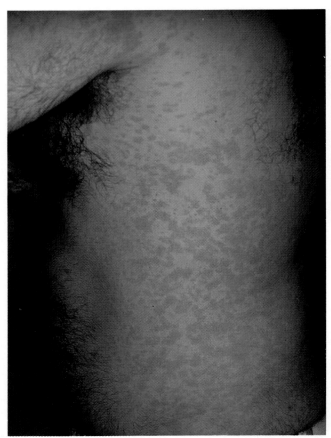

18.14
Viral exanthem.

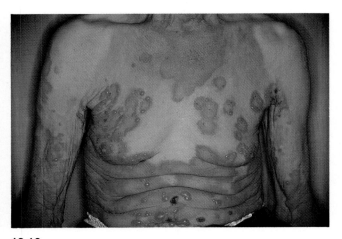

18.16
Bullous pemphigoid.[2]

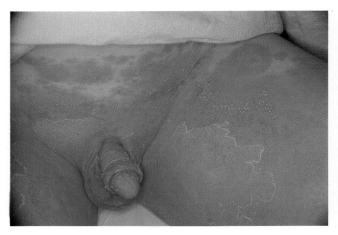

18.15
Pustular psoriasis.

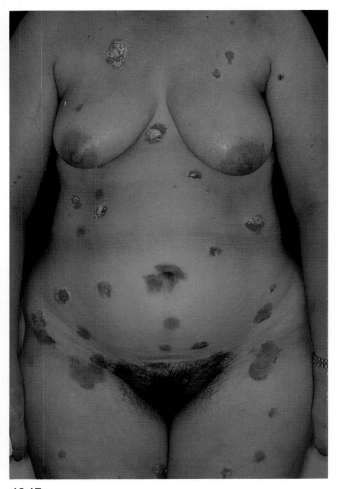

18.17
Pemphigus vulgaris.

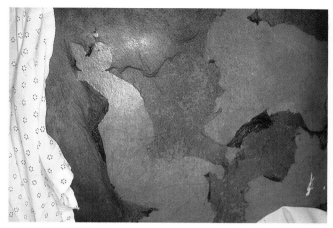

18.18
Toxic epidermal necrolysis.

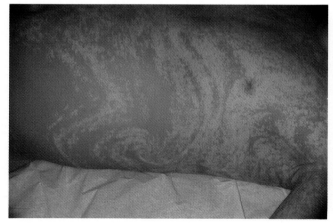

18.19
Incontinentia pigmenti.

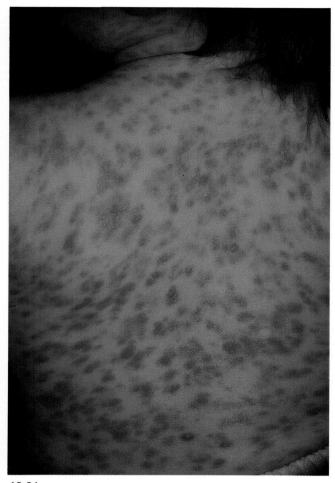

18.21
Urticaria pigmentosa.

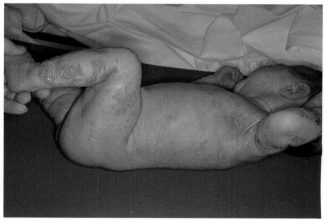

18.20
Hypomelanosis of Ito (incontinentia pigmenti achromians).

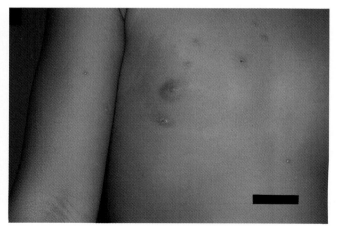

18.22
Varicella.

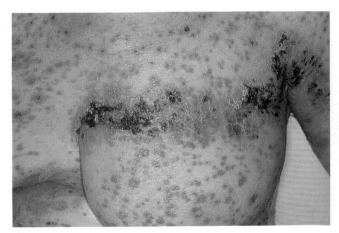

18.23
Disseminated herpes zoster.[3]

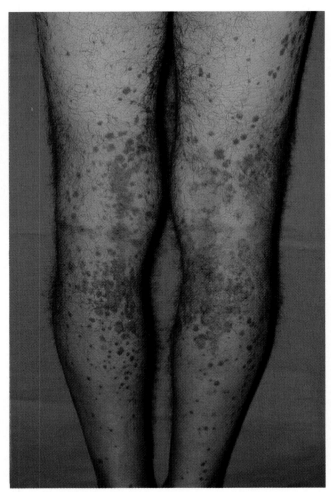

18.25
Leukocytoclastic vasculitis.[5]

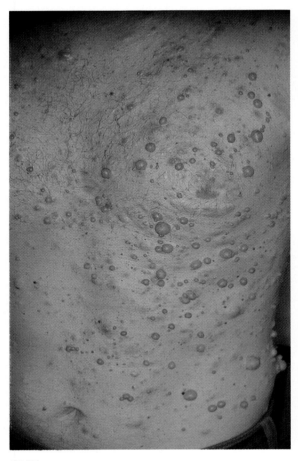

18.24
Neurofibromatosis.

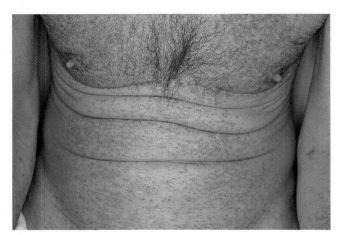

18.26
Scurvy.

The four classic ichthyoses are represented in the next four figures. There are a multitude of syndromes in which cutaneous ichthyosis is a major feature (Table XI).

TABLE XI
Characteristics of More Common Disorders of Cornification

Type	Inheritance Pattern	Onset	Cutaneous Features	Associations	Comments
Ichthyosis vulgaris	AD	3–12 mo	Fine white scales, esp. legs Palmoplantar keratoderma Seasonal variation	Atopy	Decreased granular layers and filaggrin protein
X-linked ichthyosis	X-LR	0–3 mo	Brown, adherent scales "Dirty neck" Usually normal	Corneal opacities May have genital defects	Deficiency of a sulfatase Increased epidermal cholesterol sulfate
Classic lamellar ichthyosis	AR	Usually birth: collodion	Large, platelike dark scales Ectropion, alopecia		
Nonbullous congenital ichthyosiform erythroderma	AR	Usually birth: collodion	Fine white scales Overlying variable erythema Little ectropion Alopecia		
Bullous congenital ichthyosiform erythroderma	AD	Birth	Superficial blisters, esp. in infancy Verrucous scaling, esp. at joints	Pyogenic infections	Epidermolytic hyperkeratosis on biopsy
Erythrokeratodermia variabilis	AD	Up to 3 yr	Erythematous plaques Hyperkeratotic polycyclic plaques		
Sjögren-Larsson syndrome	AR	Birth or infancy	Resembles nonbullous congenital ichthyosiform erythroderma	Spasticity Retardation Retinal degeneration Speech defects Seizures	Defect in fatty alcohol cycle
Chondrodysplasia punctata	AR AD X-D	Birth	Scaling plaques, overlying whorls, erythema, clears in first 6 mo Residual follicular atrophoderma, cicatricial alopecia	Cataracts Shortened femora, humeri Epiphyseal stippling, other skeletal changes	
Netherton's syndrome	AR	Usually birth	Serpiginous, double-edge scale (ichthyosis linearis circumflexa) Congenital ichthyosiform erythroderma Short, brittle hair (trichorrhexis invaginata)	Atopy	
Ichthyosis–brittle hair–impaired intelligence–decreased fertility–short stature (IBIDS) syndrome	AR	Birth, early infancy	Resembles nonbullous congenital ichthyosiform erythroderma Hypoplastic nails Brittle hair with trichothiodystrophy	Retardation Decreased fertility Short stature	May be photosensitive (PIBIDS)

AD, Autosomal dominant; AR, autosomal recessive; X-D, X-linked, dominant; X-LR, X-linked, recessive.

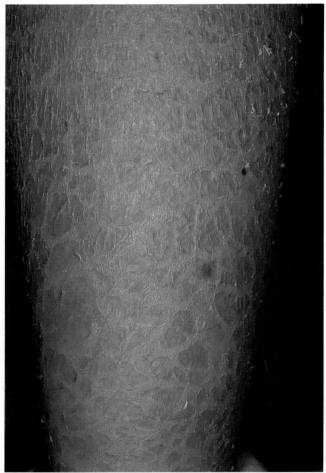

18.27
Ichthyosis vulgaris. This autosomal dominant disease is characterized by generalized, noninflammatory, fine white scale.[2]

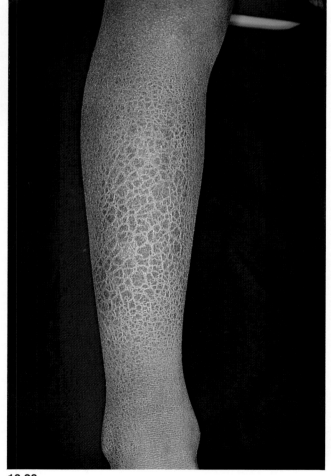

18.28
X-linked ichthyosis. An X-linked recessive disorder. This patient's mother is probably an unaffected carrier.[6]

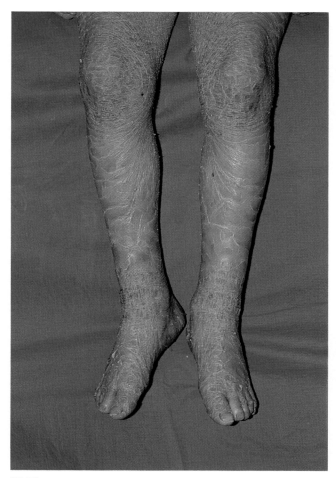

18.29
Lamellar ichthyosis. An autosomal recessive disorder in which there are thick scales.

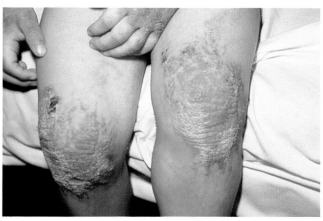

18.30
Bullous congenital ichthyosiform erythroderma (epidermolytic hyperkeratosis). An autosomal dominant disorder with coarse verrucous scales. There is a predilection for flexural surfaces.

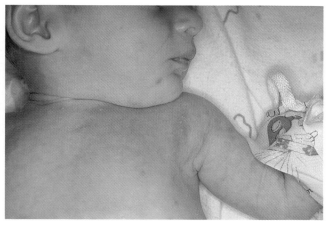

18.31
Erythema toxicum of the newborn.

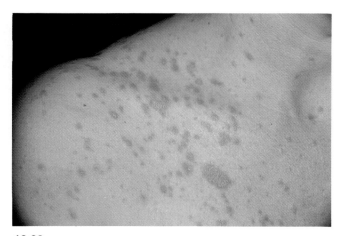

18.32
Pityriasis rosea.

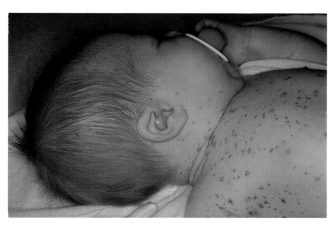

18.33
Histiocytosis X.

DISORDERS WITH A PHOTODISTRIBUTION

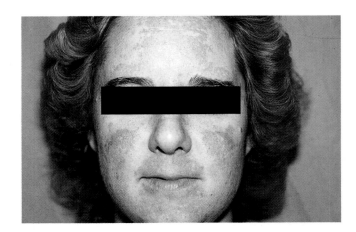

19.1
Melasma.

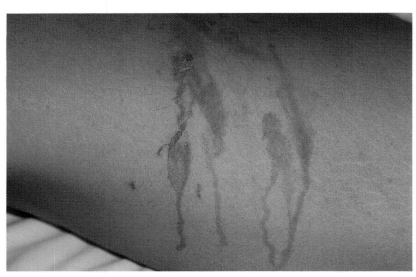

A

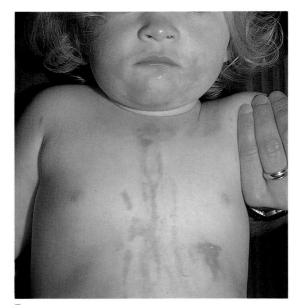

B

19.2
A, B, Phototoxic contact dermatitis (berloque dermatitis).

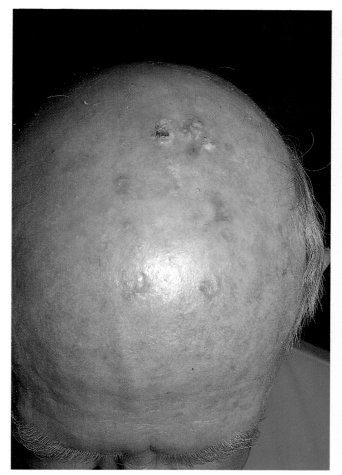

19.3
Actinic keratoses.

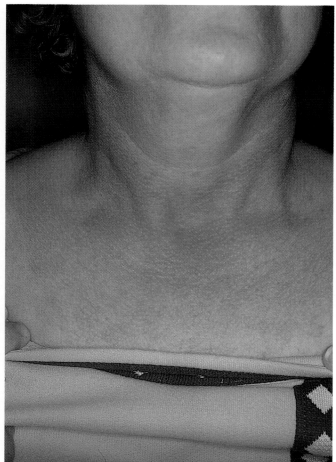

19.5
Poikiloderma of Civatte.

19.4
Sunburn reaction.

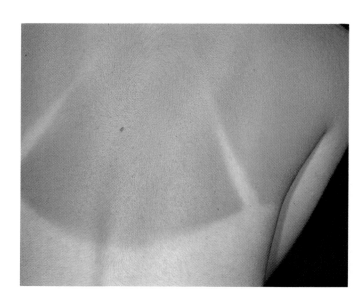

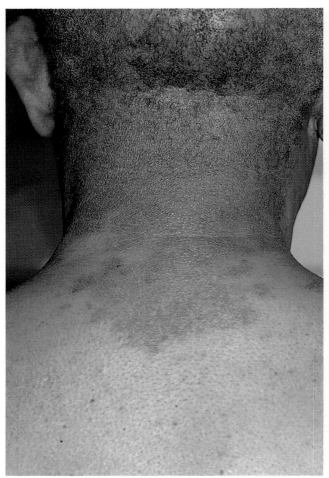

19.6
Photosensitivity dermatitis due to thiazide ingestion.

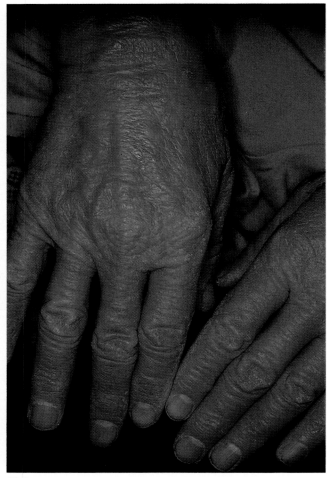

19.8
Actinic reticuloid. Persistent photodermatitis in older men.

19.7
Persistent light reaction. These patients continue to react to ultraviolet light despite removal of the photosensitizer.

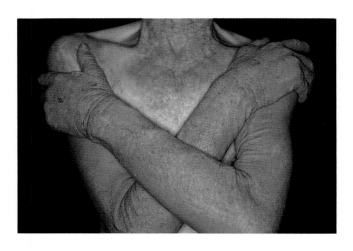

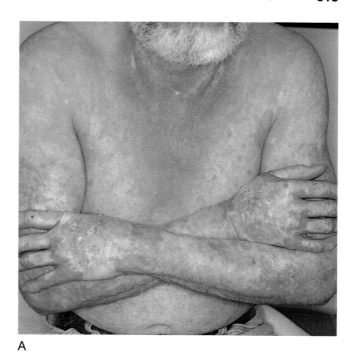

A

19.9
A, B, Subacute cutaneous lupus erythematosus, papulo-squamous variant.

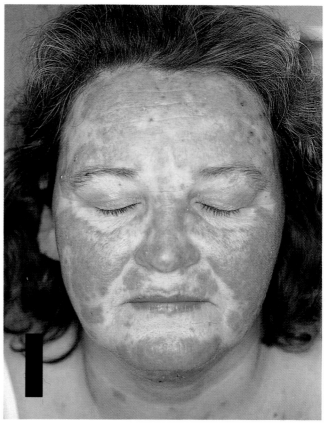

B

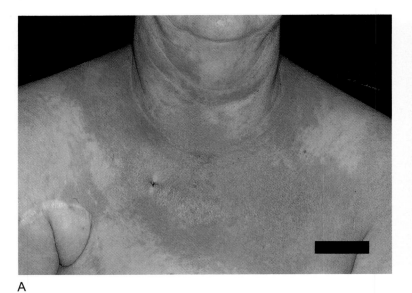

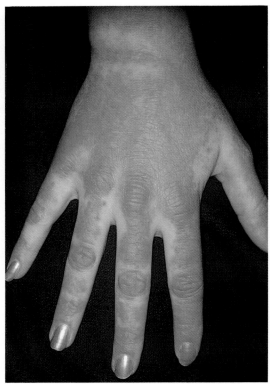

19.10
Dermatomyositis. Poikiloderma in the "v" of the neck *(A)*. Note the sparing of the interdigitial web spaces *(B)*.

A

B

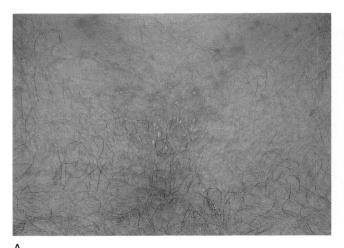

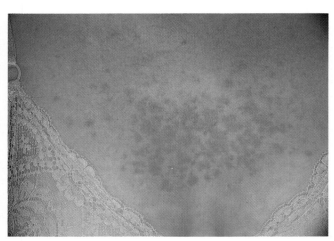

A

B

19.11
A, B, Polymorphous light eruption.

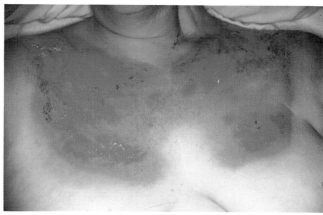

19.12
Methotrexate-induced sunburn recall.[3]

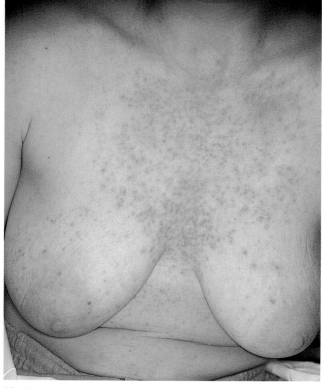

19.14
Darier's disease.

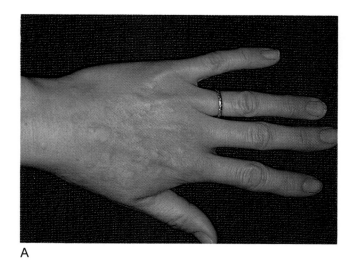

A

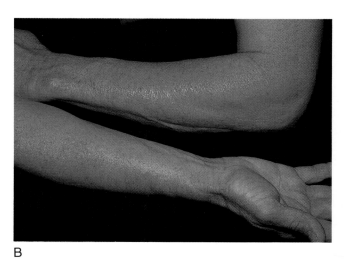

B

19.13
A, B, Lichen planus actinicus.

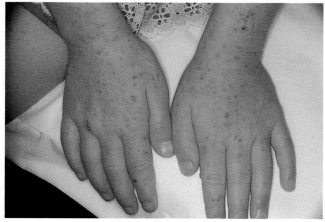

19.15
Actinic prurigo.

INTERTRIGINOUS AND GENITAL PROBLEMS

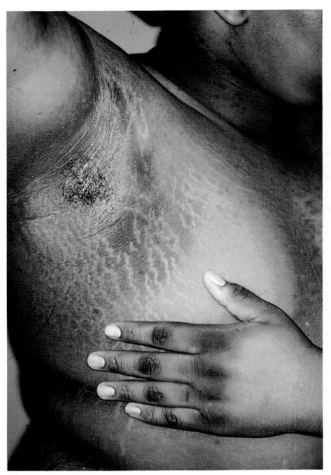

20.1
Acanthosis nigricans.

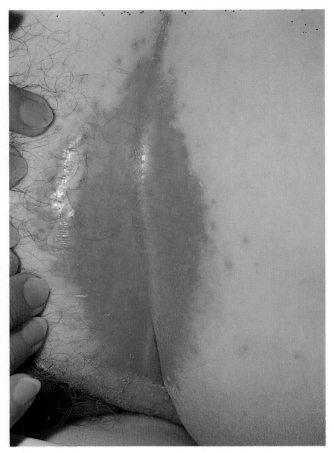

20.2
Candida infection in the intergluteal fold.

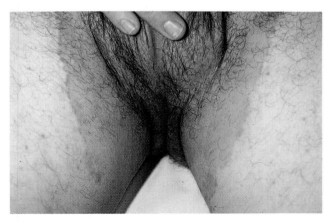

20.3
Tinea cruris.

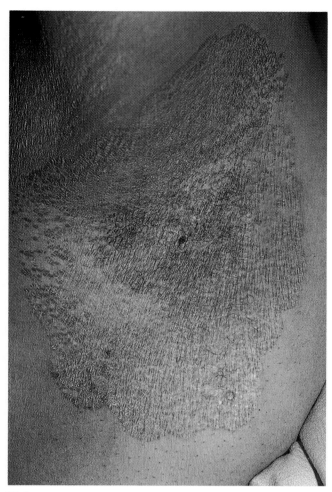

20.4
Erythrasma.

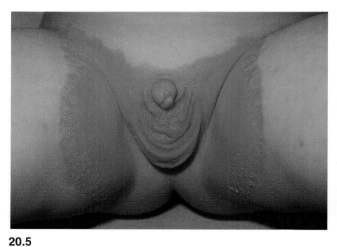

20.5
Seborrheic dermatitis.

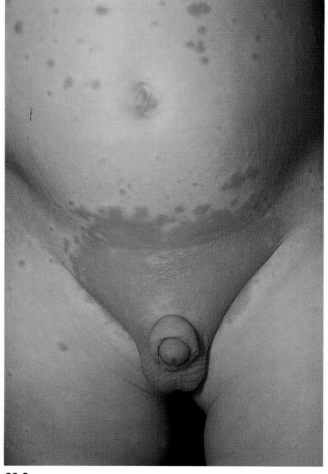

20.6
"Napkin" psoriasis.

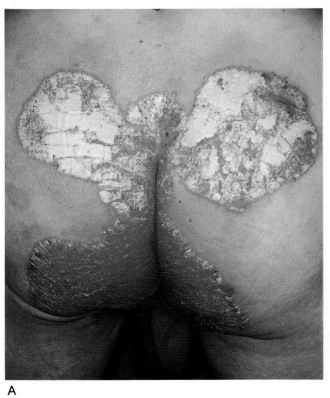

A

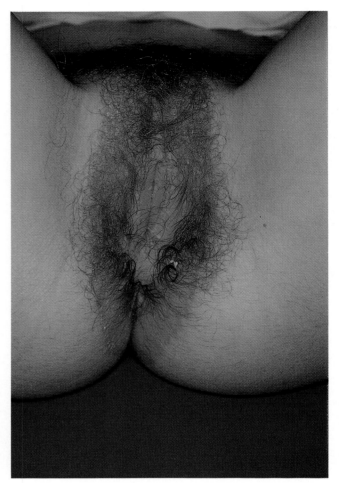

B

20.7
A, B, Psoriasis.

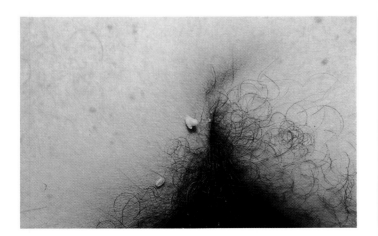

20.8
Skin tag (acrochordon).

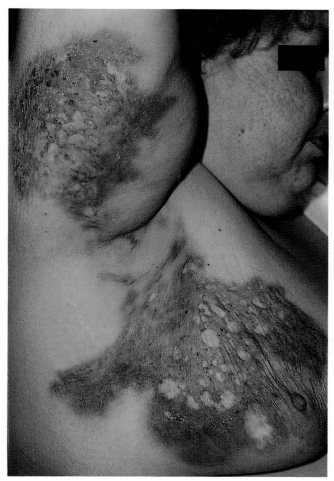

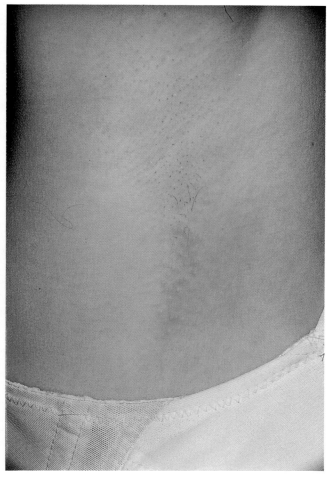

20.9
Hidradenitis suppurativa. An inflammatory condition of the apocrine glands.

20.10
Fox-Fordyce disease (apocrine miliaria).

20.11
Hailey-Hailey disease (benign familial chronic pemphigus).

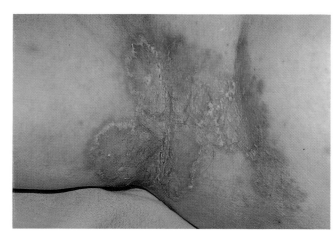

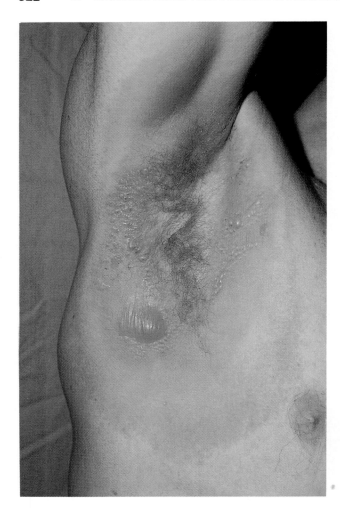

20.12
Contact dermatitis.

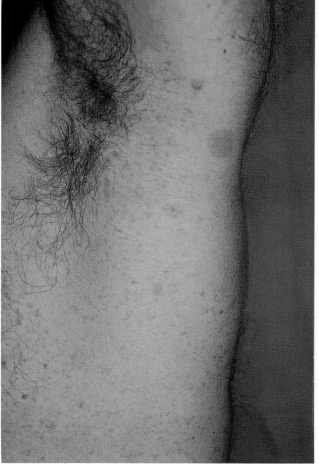

20.13
Axillary freckling (Crowe's sign) in neurofibromatosis.

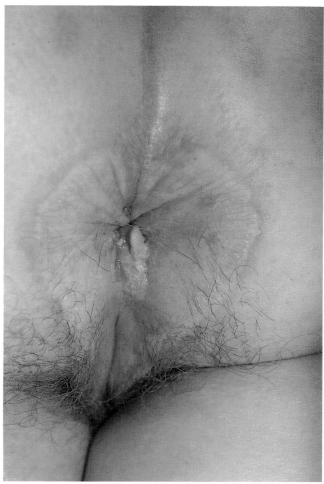

20.14
Lichen sclerosus et atrophicus.

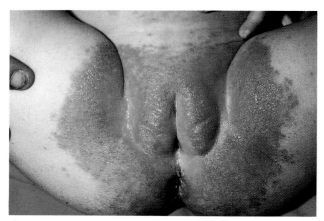

20.16
Diaper dermatitis.

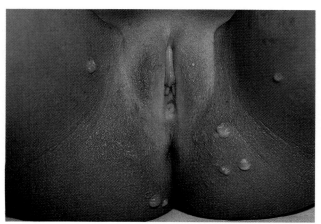

20.17
Bullous impetigo.

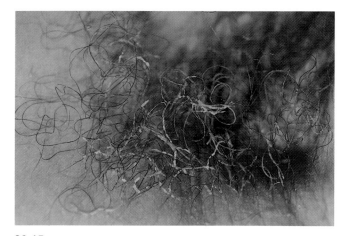

20.15
Trichomycosis axillaris. This yellow-orange crust on the hair is due to infection with *Corynebacterium tenuis*.

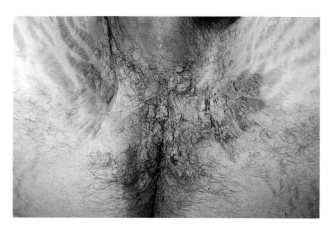

20.18
Pemphigus vegetans. A vegetative variant of pemphigus vulgaris.

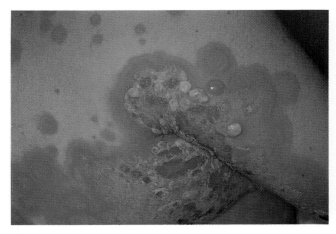

20.19
Bullous pemphigoid.

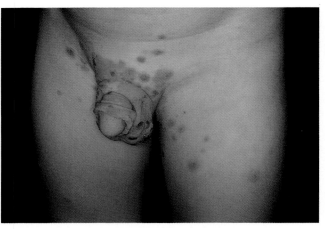

20.21
Chronic bullous disease of childhood (linear IgA disease).

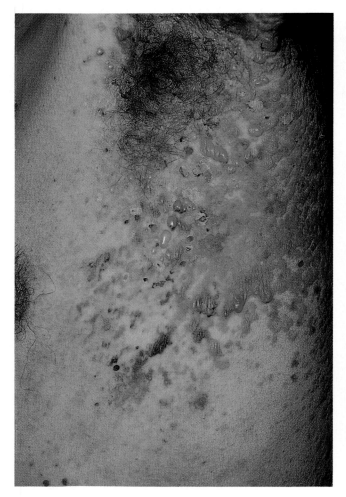

20.20
Linear IgA bullous dermatosis.

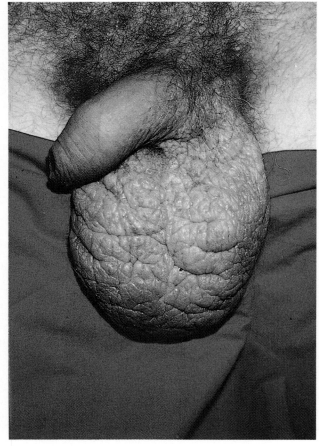

20.22
Lichen simplex chronicus of the scrotum.

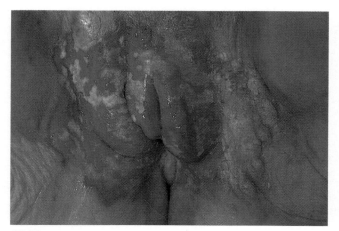

20.23
Extramammary Paget's disease. Frequently but not always associated with an underlying carcinoma.

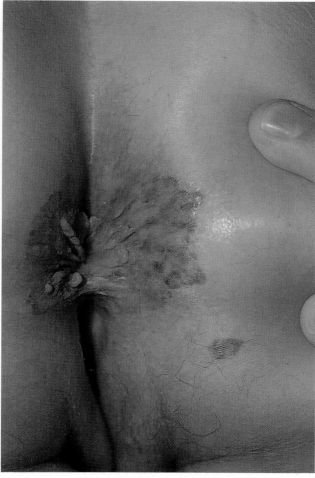

20.25
Perianal Bowen's disease (in situ squamous cell carcinoma).

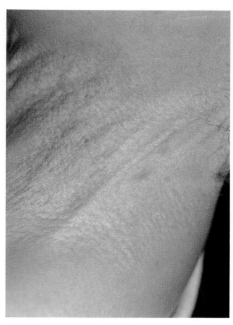

20.24
Pseudoxanthoma elasticum.

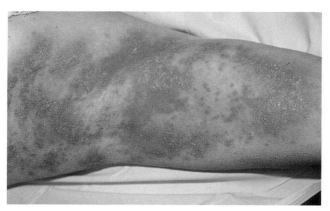

20.26
Subcorneal pustular dermatosis.

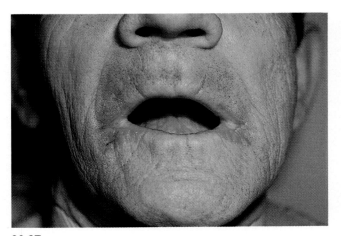

20.27
Perlèche.

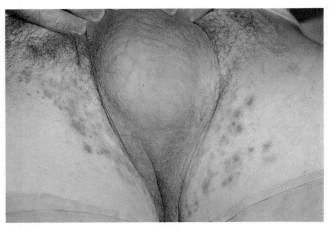

20.29
Necrolytic migratory erythema of the glucagonoma syndrome.

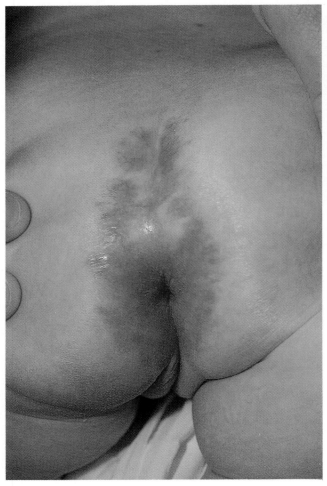

20.28
Histiocytosis X.

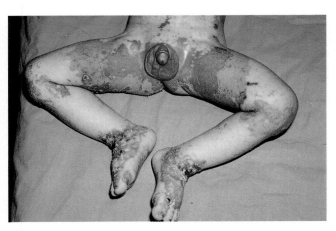

20.30
Acrodermatitis enteropathica.

GENITAL LESIONS

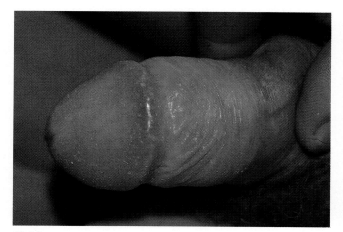

20.31
Candida balanitis.

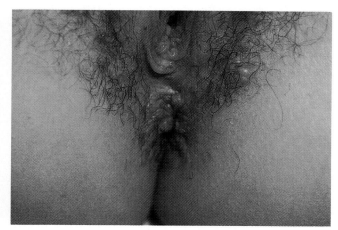

20.34
Bowenoid papulosis.

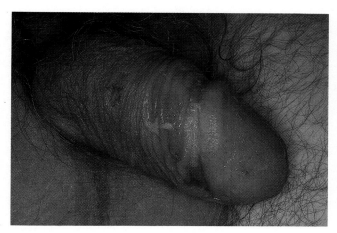

20.32
Fixed drug eruption.

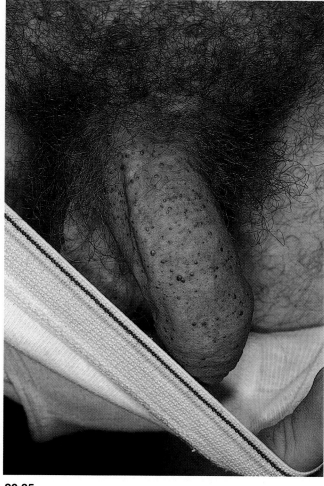

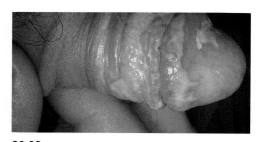

20.33
Balanitis xerotica obliterans (lichen sclerosus et atrophicus).

20.35
Angiokeratoma corporis diffusum universale (Fabry's disease).

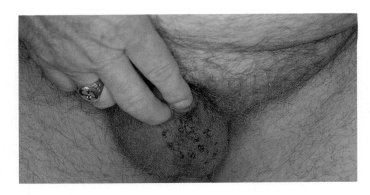

20.36
Angiokeratoma of Fordyce.

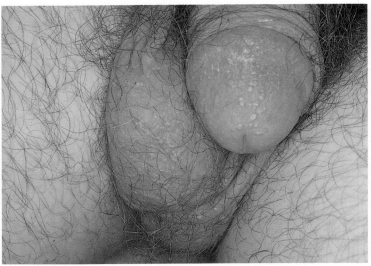

A
20.37
A, *B*, Lichen planus.

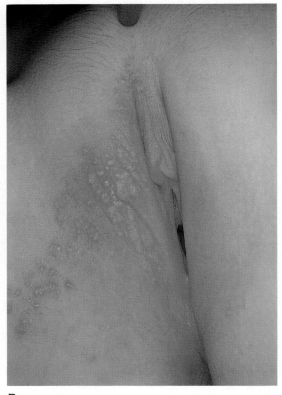

B

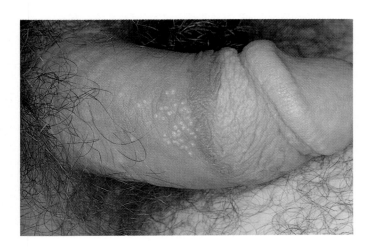

20.38
Molluscum contagiosum.

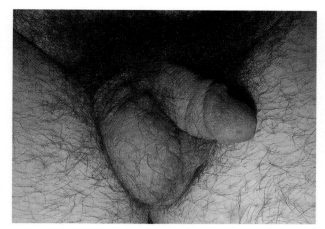

20.39
Scabies.

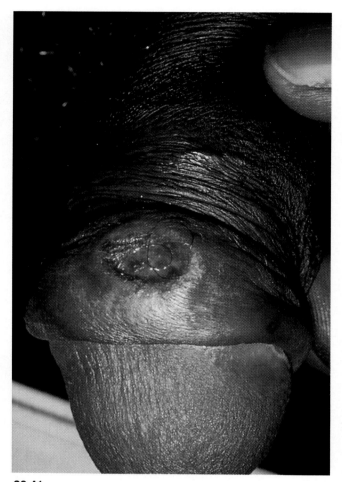

20.41
Chancre of primary syphilis.

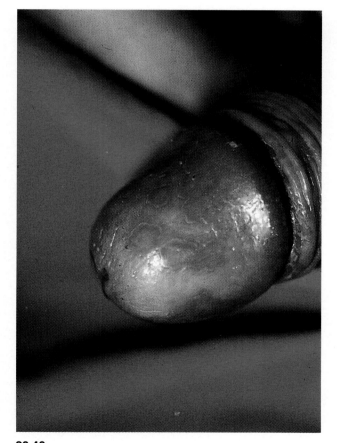

20.40
Circinate balanitis in Reiter's disease.

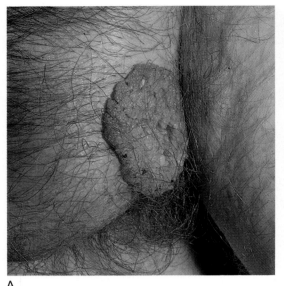

A

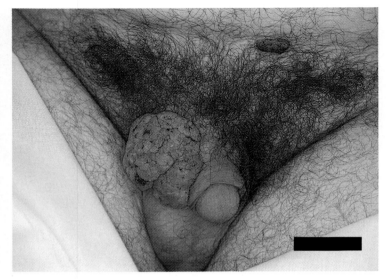

B

20.42
A, B, Condyloma acuminatum.

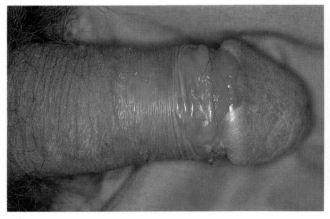

20.43
Erythroplasia of Queyrat. In situ squamous cell carcinoma similar to Bowen's disease.

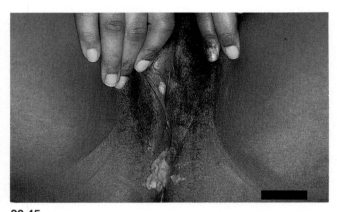

20.45
Vulvar pyoderma gangrenosum.

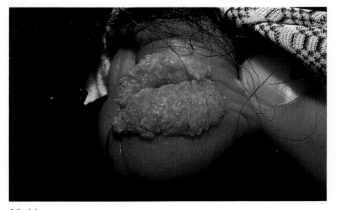

20.44
Verrucous carcinoma of the penis (Buschke-Löwenstein).

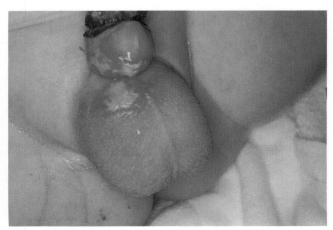

20.46
Penile pyoderma gangrenosum.

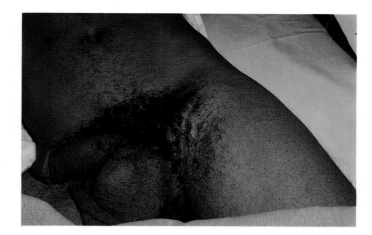

20.47
Lymphogranuloma venereum.

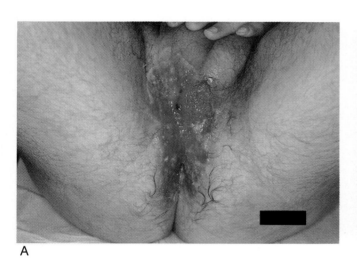

A

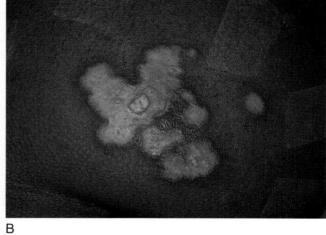

B

20.48
Atypical herpes simplex in an HIV-positive man *(A)* and in a renal transplant recipient *(B)*.

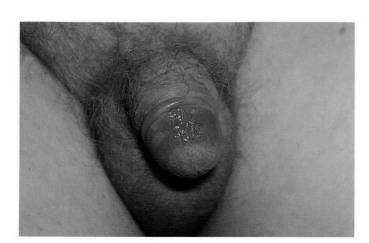

20.49
Plasma cell balanitis (Zoon's).

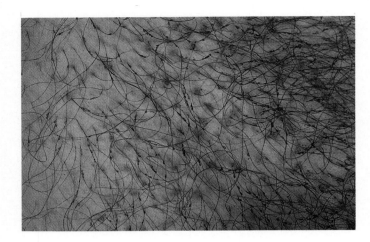

20.50
Pediculosis pubis.

LESIONS ON THE HANDS AND FEET*

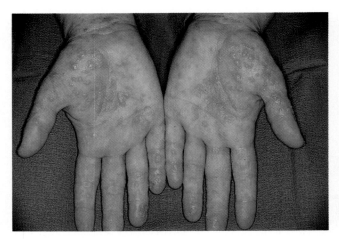

21.1
Dyshidrotic eczema.[2]

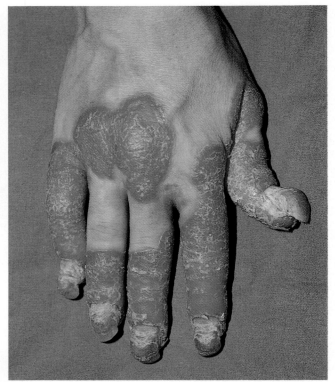

A

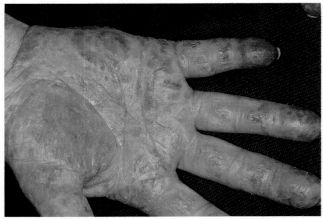

21.2
Psoriasiform dermatitis.

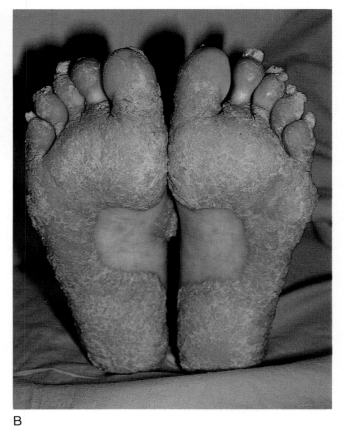

B
21.3
A, B, Psoriasis vulgaris.

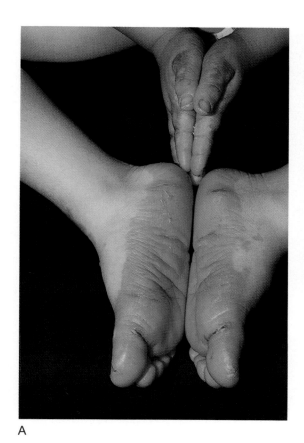

A

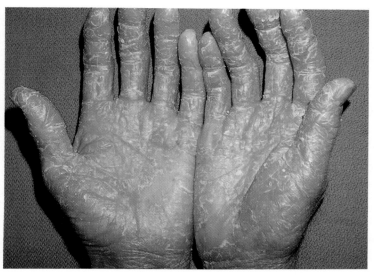

B

21.4
A, B, Pityriasis rubra pilaris.

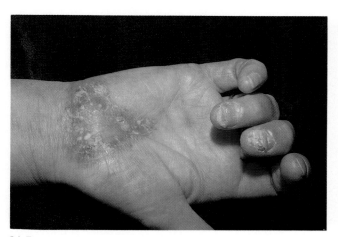

21.5
Acrodermatitis continua. Chronic, pustular dermatitis with sharp dermarcation.

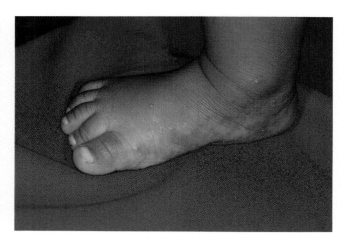

21.6
Acropustulosis of infancy.

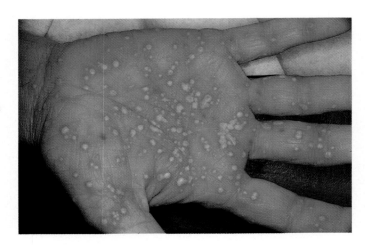

21.7
Pustular palmoplantar psoriasis.

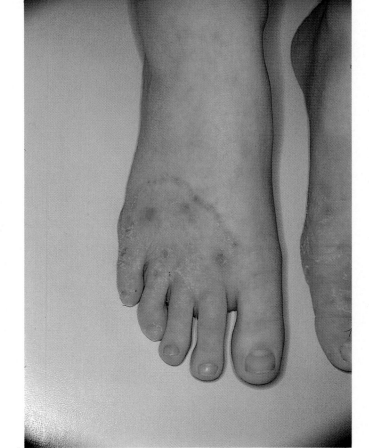

21.8
Tinea pedis.

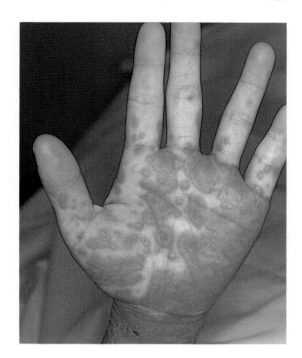

21.9
Erythema multiforme.

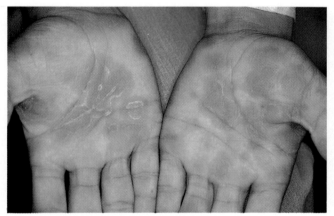

21.10
Secondary syphilis.[10]

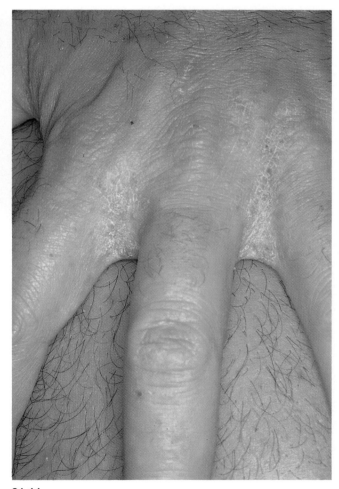

21.11
Scabies.

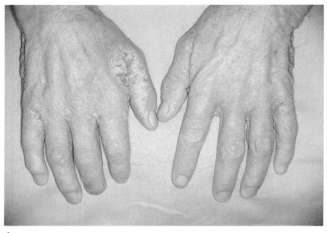

A

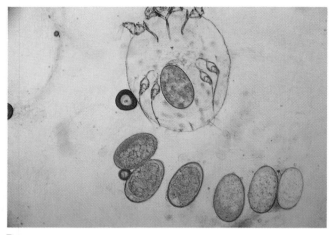

B

21.12
A[2], Norwegian (crusted) scabies. *B,* Skin scraping from a patient with scabies.

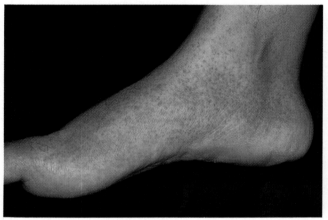

21.13
Rocky Mountain spotted fever.[6]

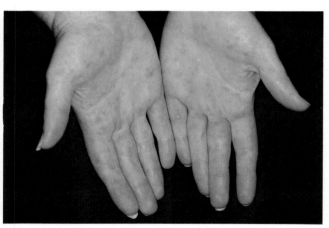

21.15
Hand-foot-and-mouth disease.

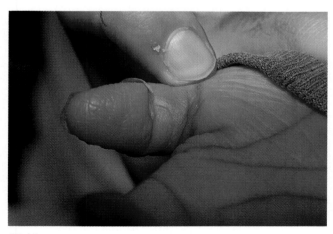

21.14
Kawasaki's disease.[13]

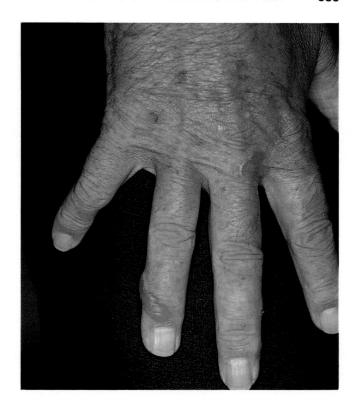

21.16
Epidermolysis bullosa acquisita.

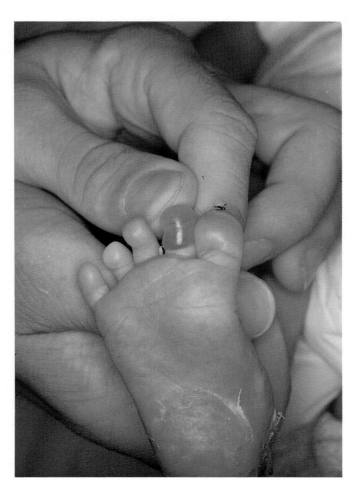

21.17
Epidermolysis bullosa simplex.

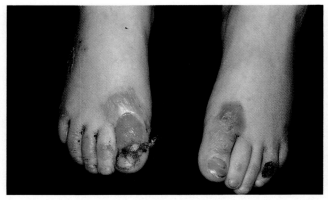

21.18
Epidermolysis bullosa dystrophica, dominant.

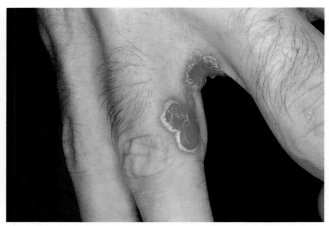

21.21
Reiter's disease.

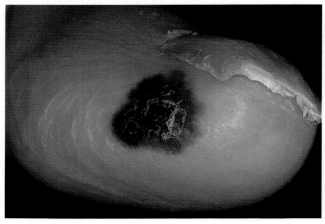

21.19
Acrolentiginous malignant melanoma.[2]

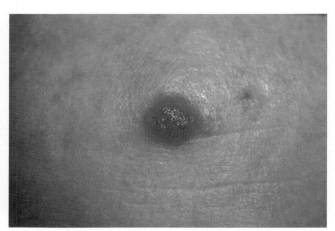

21.22
Orf.

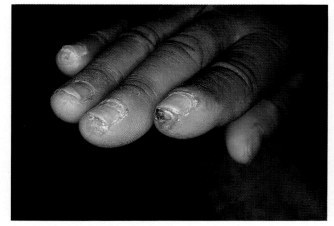

21.20
Scleroderma. This patient has severe Raynaud's phenomenon with ulceration of the distal fingertip.

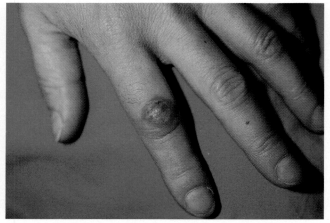

21.23
Milker's nodule.

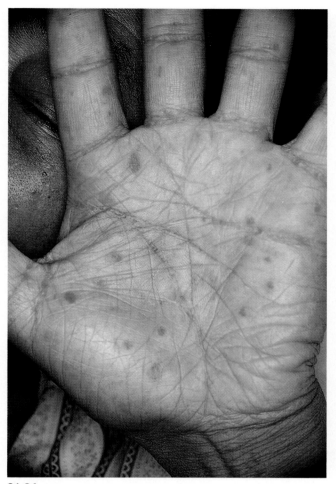

21.24
Hereditary hemorrhagic telangiectasia.

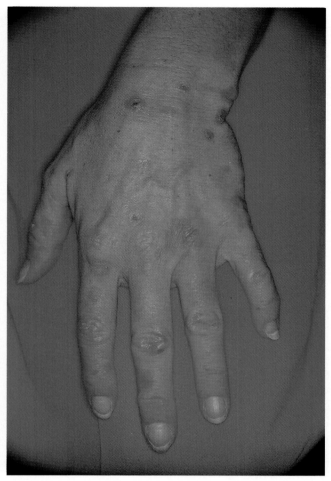

21.25
Porphyria cutanea tarda.

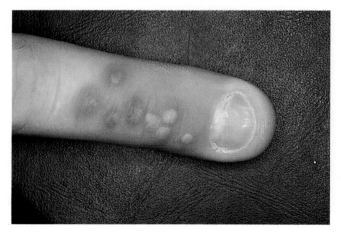

21.26
Herpetic whitlow.

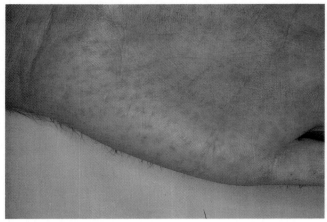

21.27
Fabry's disease.

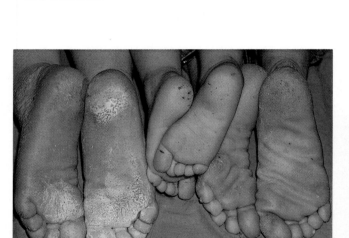

21.28
Palmoplantar keratoderma, Unna-Thost variant. Autosomal dominant trait in grandfather, father, and son.

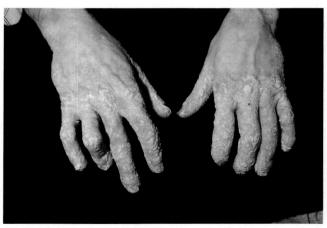

21.29
Vohwinkel's palmoplantar keratoderma (mutilating keratoderma) is inherited as an autosomal dominant trait.

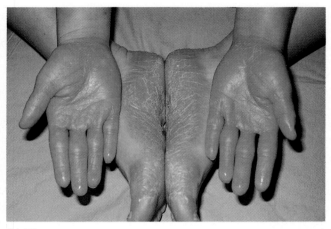

21.30
Papillon-Lefèvre syndrome (palmoplantar keratoderma with periodontitis). This is an autosomal recessive syndrome that includes keratoderma, periodontoclasia, and calcification of the dura.[5]

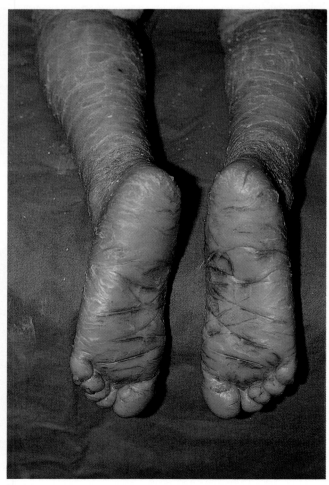

21.31
Lamellar ichthyosis.[5]

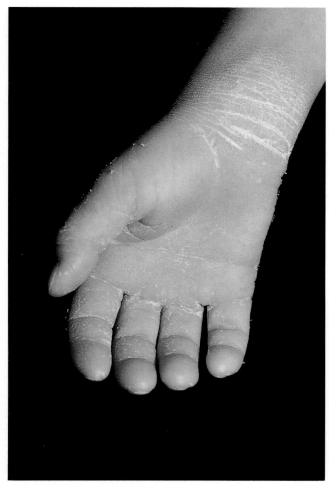

21.32
Bullous congenital ichthyosiform erythroderma (epidermolytic hyperkeratosis).

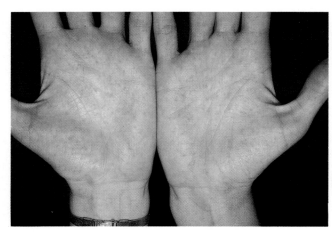

21.33
Basal cell nevus syndrome.

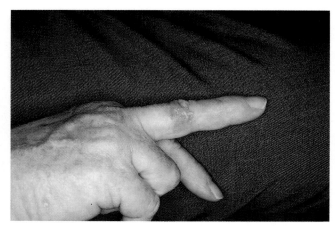

21.34
Bowen's disease.

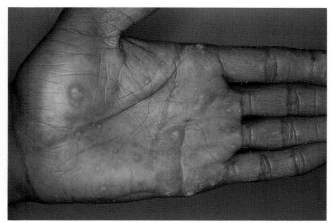

21.35
Arsenical keratoses.

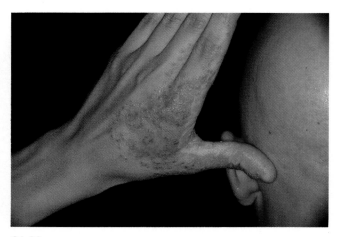

21.36
Chronic mucocutaneous candidiasis as part of a polyglandular syndrome with insulin-resistant diabetes mellitus, hypothyroidism, and alopecia totalis.

NAIL DISORDERS

These disorders can be divided into those that affect certain parts of the nail. Thus, they can be separated into (1) those that affect the matrix, (2) those that affect the nail bed, and (3) those that affect the nail folds or surrounding tissue. Disorders of the matrix may be further subdivided into those that destroy the matrix, those that cause disruption or cessation of growth (atrophy), those that are associated with excess thickness (hypertrophy), and those in which the keratinization is abnormal.

DISORDERS OF THE NAIL PLATE

Absence or Hypoplasia of Nails

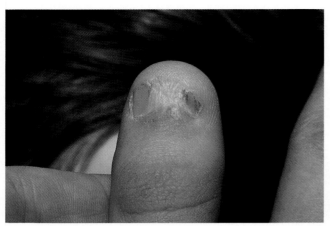

22.1
Nail-patella syndrome. An autosomal dominant disease characterized by absence or hypoplasia of the nails and the patella and the presence of iliac horns. Nephrosis is common in these patients and can progress to renal insufficiency.

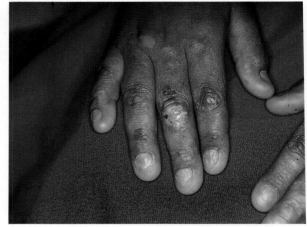

22.3
Generalized benign atrophic epidermolysis bullosa. All forms of junctional epidermolysis bullosa are associated with nail abnormalities.

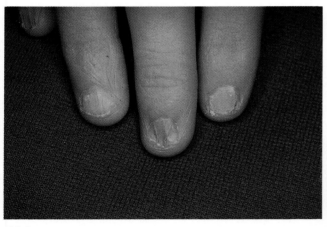

22.2
Dyskeratosis congenita.

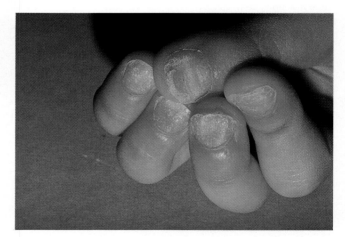

22.4
Twenty-nail dystrophy. This may be a variant of lichen planus.

Onycholysis (Separation of the Nail Plate from the Nail Bed)

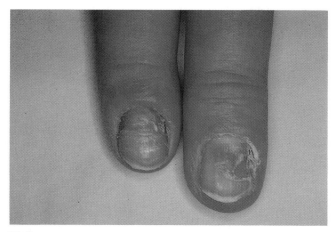

22.5
Candida albicans infection.[2]

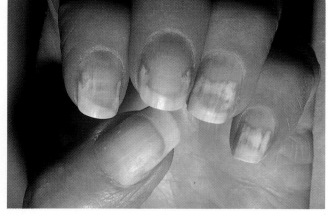

22.8
Drug-induced onycholysis. This was a common finding in patients treated with benoxaprofen (which has been removed from the market).

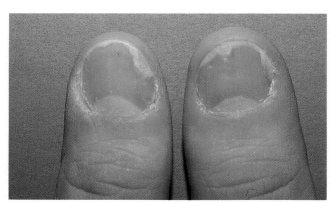

22.6
Dermatophyte infection.[2]

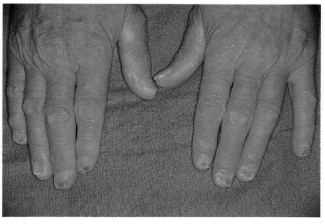

22.7
Psoriasis.

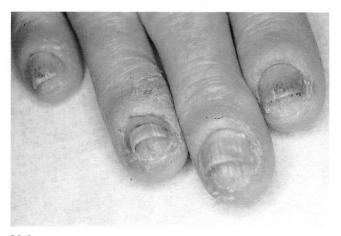

22.9
Onycholysis secondary to false "solar" nails.

Pits and Grooves

These suggest a disorder in growth of the matrix.

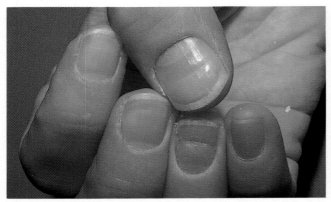

22.10
Beau's lines. This patient had major surgery 5 months previously.

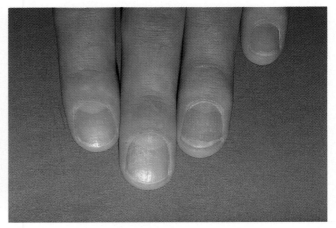

22.12
Alopecia areata.

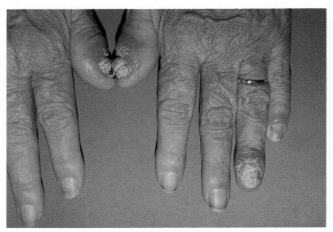

A

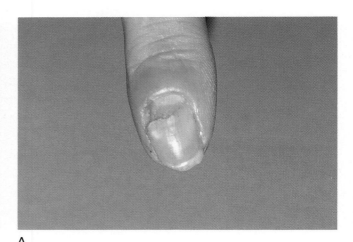

A

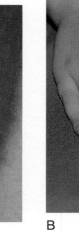

B

22.11
A, B, Psoriasis.

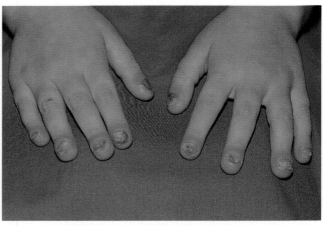

B

22.13
A, B, Candidal paronychia. *B,* Occurring in a patient with chronic mucocutaneous candidiasis.

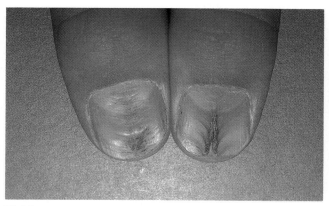

22.14
Habit tic deformity due to continued trauma at the base of the nail plate.

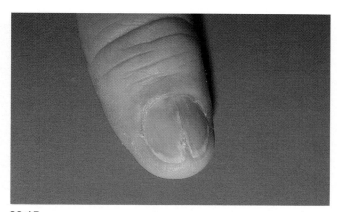

22.15
Median nail dystrophy.

Color Changes

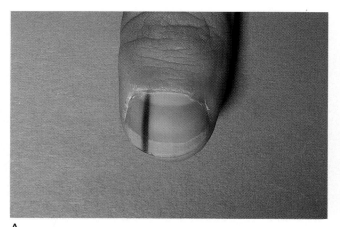

A

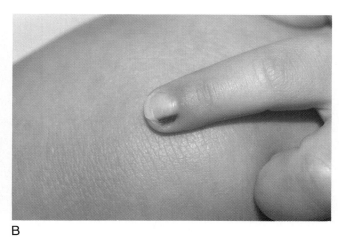

B

22.16
A, *B*, Junctional nevus of the nail bed.

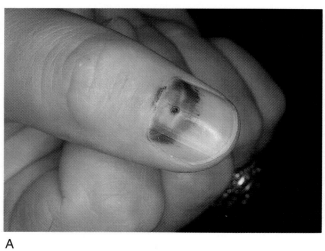

A

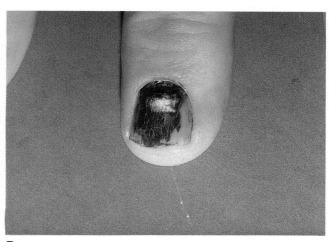

B

22.17
A, *B*, Traumatic injury with hemorrhage.

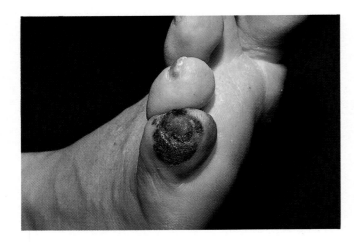

22.18
Malignant melanoma. Note that the pigment diffuses into the surrounding tissue.

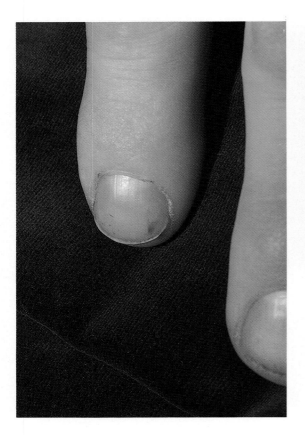

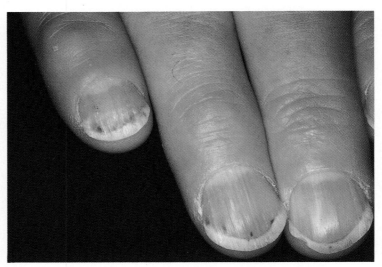

B

22.19
Splinter hemorrhages. *A*, In subacute bacterial endocarditis. *B*, In a patient with leukocytoclastic vasculitis.

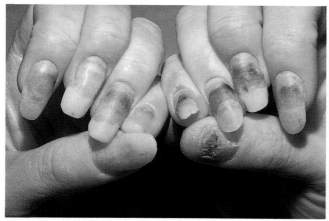

22.20
Pseudomonas infection of the nails. Onycholysis with green-black malodorous debris.

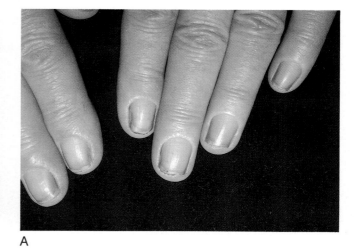

A

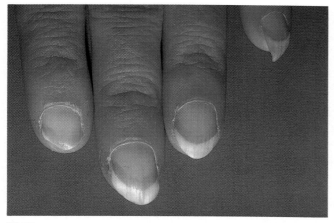

22.21
Half-and-half nails in a patient with chronic renal failure.

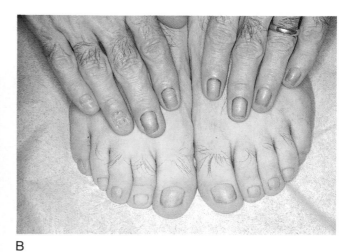

B

22.23
A, B, Yellow nail syndrome. These patients are commonly found to have pulmonary disease.

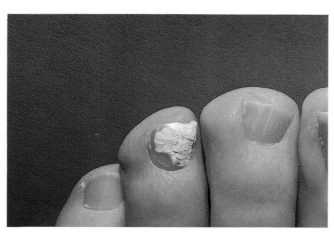

22.22
Infection with *Trichophyton mentagrophytes*.

Thickening of the Nail Plate

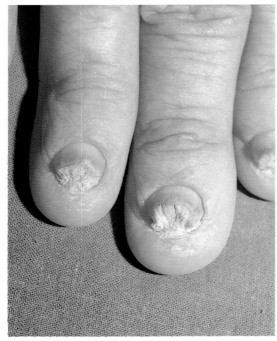

A

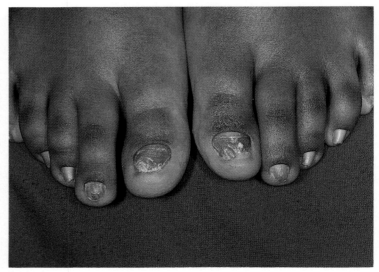

B

22.24
A, *B*, Pachyonychia congenita.

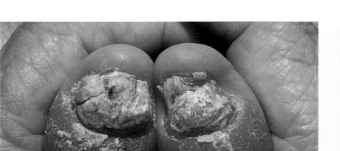

22.25
Psoriasis vulgaris.

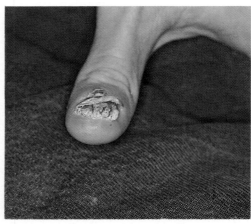

22.26
Reiter's syndrome.

Thinning of the Nail Plate

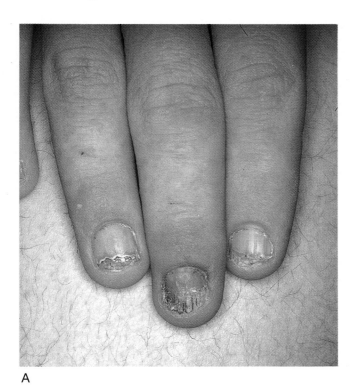

A

22.27
Darier's disease. *A*, Wedge-shaped onycholysis. *B*, With
typical keratotic papules on the skin.

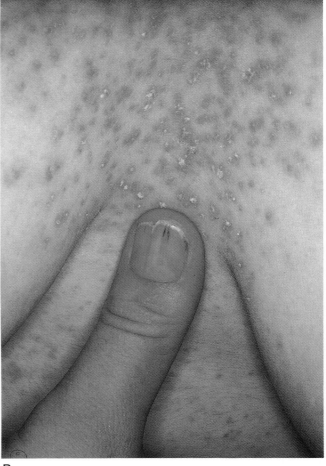

B

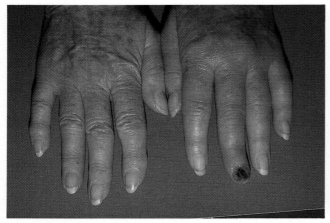

22.28
Raynaud's phenomenon in a patient with scleroderma.

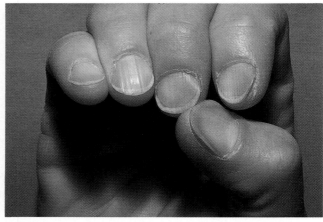

22.29
Koilonychia. May be seen with iron deficiency anemia.

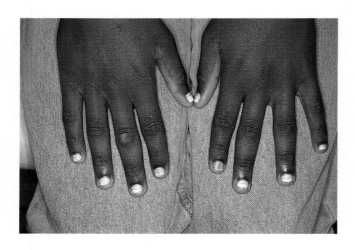

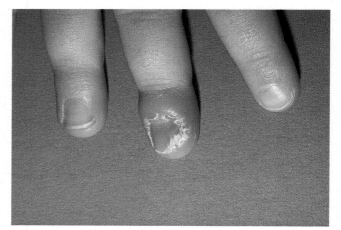

22.30
Leukonychia.

DISEASES OF THE NAIL FOLD

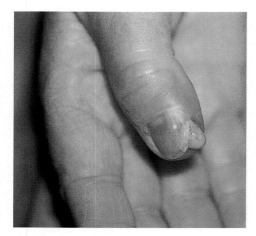

22.31
Acute bacterial paronychia. *Staphylococcus aureus* was cultured from this patient.

22.32
Candida albicans paronychia.

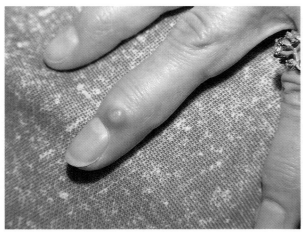

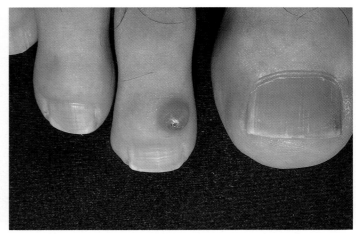

A

B

22.33

A, B, Mucinous pseudocyst or myxoid cyst.

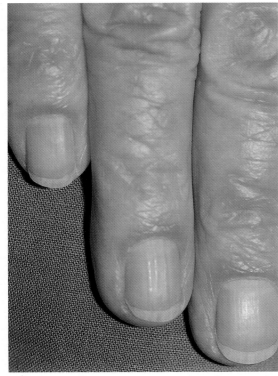

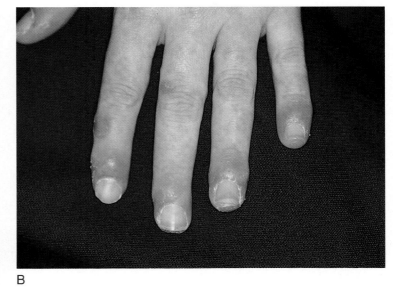

A

B

22.34

A, B, Periungual erythema and telangiectasias—lupus erythematosus.

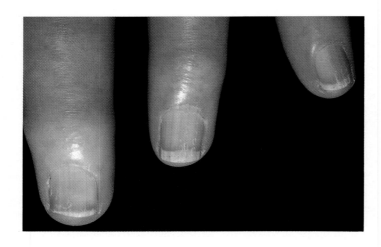

22.35
Periungual erythema and telangiectasias—scleroderma.

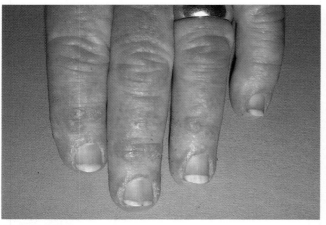

22.36
Periungual erythema and telangiectasias—dermatomyositis.

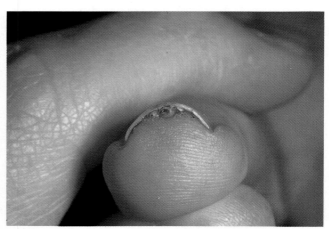

22.38
Subungual fibroma in tuberous sclerosis.[9]

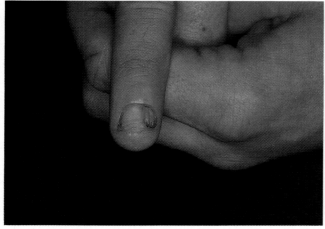

A

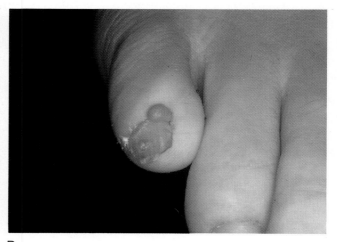

B

22.37
A, B, Periungual fibroma in tuberous sclerosis.

MISCELLANEOUS

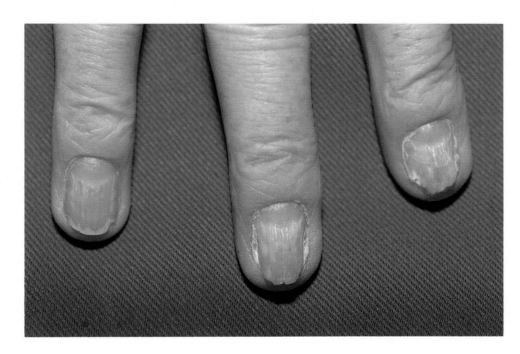

22.39
Nail dystrophy of Cronkhite-Canada syndrome.

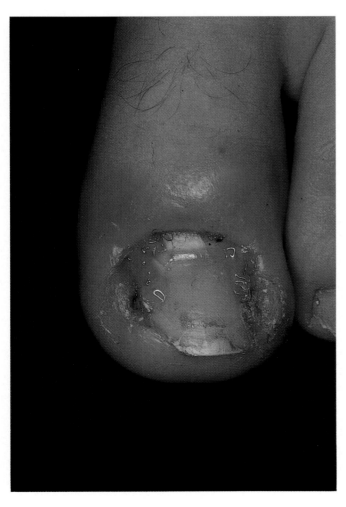

22.40
Ingrown toenail.[6]

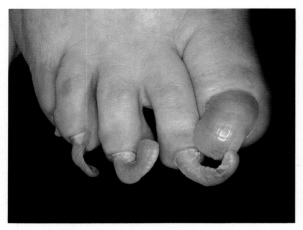

22.41
Onychogryphosis.

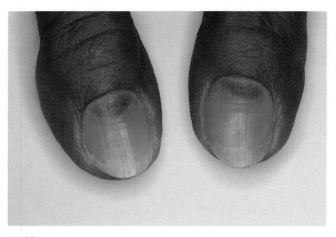

22.42
Pigmentation of the lunulae in a patient on psoralen plus ultraviolet A (PUVA) therapy.

CHAPTER 23

HAIR AND SCALP DISORDERS

TABLE XII
Diseases of the Hair and Scalp

1. Developmental defects or inherited disorders
   Aplasia cutis congenita
   Nevus sebaceus and epidermal nevi
2. Infections
   Fungal
   Bacterial
3. Neoplastic
4. Physical or chemical agents
5. Inflammatory dermatoses
   Lupus erythematosus
   Lichen planopilaris
   Sarcoidosis
   Scleroderma
   Epidermolysis bullosa acquisita
   Alopecia mucinosa
   Folliculitis decalvans
   Dissecting cellulitis

Modified from Rook A, Dawber RPR: Diseases of the Hair and Scalp. Blackwell Scientific, Oxford, 1982.

LOSS OF HAIR

Congenital Disorders with Normal Hair

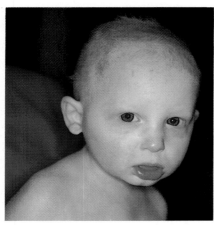

23.1
Typical facies of a boy with hypohidrotic ectodermal dysplasia. Note the full pouty lower lip and thin upper lip, the flat malar areas, the mild periorbital hyperpigmentation, the broad forehead, the sparse hair, and the abnormal ear.

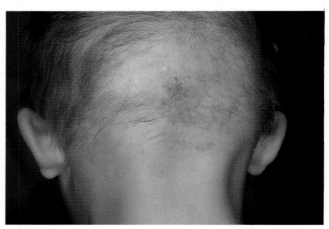

23.2
Hypohidrotic ectodermal dysplasia. Usually inherited as an X-linked recessive disorder. Patients have abnormal facies, decreased sweat and mucous glands, and sparse hair.

Congenital Disorders with Abnormal Hair

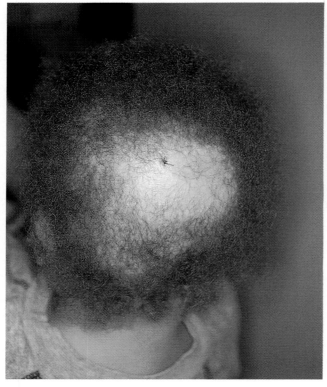

23.3
Monilethrix. The hair appears beaded in this autosomal dominant disorder.

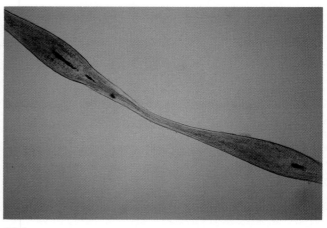

23.4
Typical hair pluck of monilethrix.

23.5
Pili torti. The hair is tortuous in this autosomal dominant disorder. Associated findings such as mental retardation, keratosis pilaris, corneal opacities, and skeletal abnormalities may occur in some patients. Patients with Menkes' syndrome have pili torti, hypopigmentation, temperature instability, seizures, and abnormal copper transport.

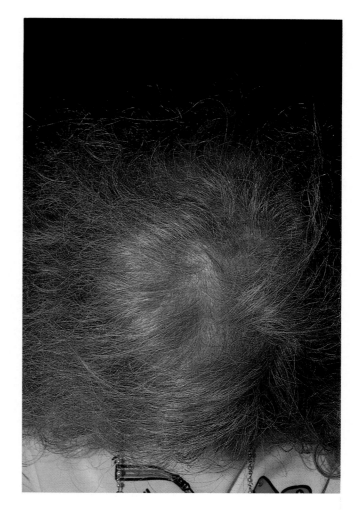

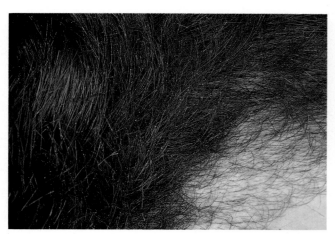

23.6
Trichorrhexis nodosa. The hair has brushlike deformities.

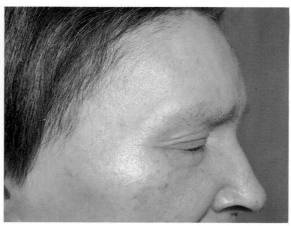

23.7
Netherton's syndrome. The hair shaft abnormality is known as trichorrhexis invaginata and is represented by a "ball in socket" appearance. This autosomal recessive disorder combines the hair shaft abnormality with ichthyosis linearis circumflexa or ichthyosiform erythroderma and atopic dermatitis.

Acquired Nonscarring Hair Loss

TABLE XIII Nonscarring Alopecias	
Androgenetic alopecia (pattern baldness) Congenital hereditary syndromes Alopecia areata Telogen effluvium Endocrinologic diseases	Infections Fungal Syphilitic Traumatic

Modified from Rook A, Dawber RPR: Diseases of the Hair and Scalp. Blackwell Scientific, Oxford, 1982.

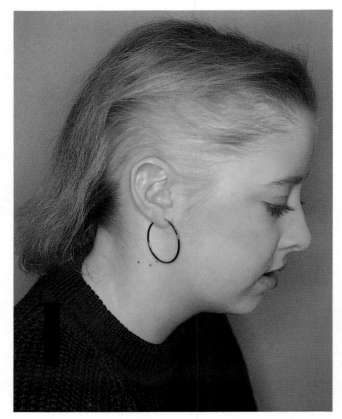

23.8
Telogen effluvium in a patient with systemic lupus erythematosus. The loss of hair occurred 2 months after an acute systemic flare-up.

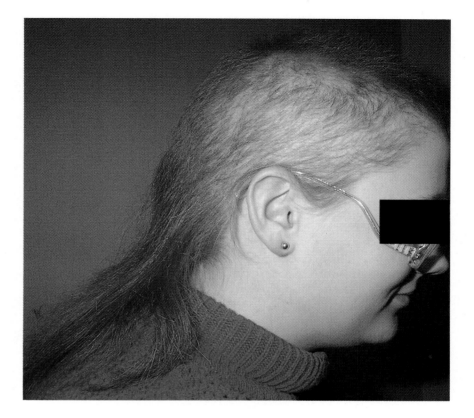

23.9
Trichotillomania. This patient manipulates and twists her hair repeatedly, resulting in breakage.

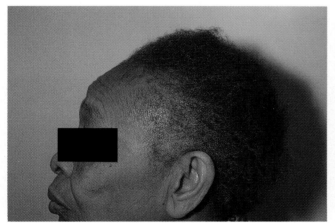

23.10
Traction alopecia from tight braiding and use of a hot comb.

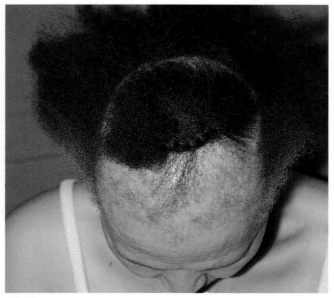

23.11
Traction alopecia.[5]

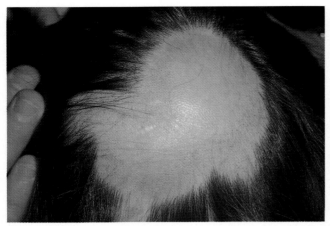

23.12
Alopecia areata. An immunologically mediated loss of hair. The cause is unknown.

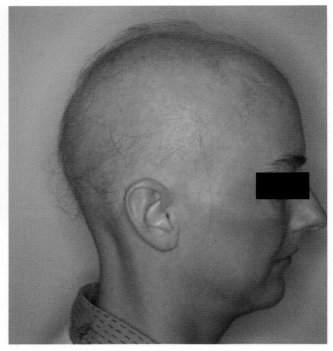

23.14
Alopecia totalis.

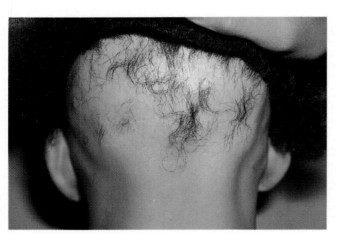

23.13
Ophiasis. A pattern of alopecia areata that involves the hair margin from above the ears to the nape of the neck.

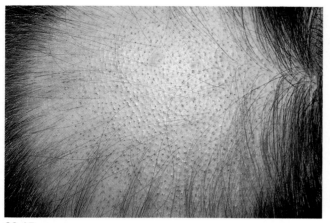

23.15
Tinea capitis from *Trichophyton tonsurans* ("black-dot" ringworm).

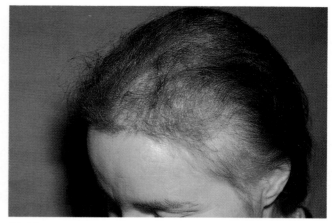

23.16
Male pattern baldness (androgenetic alopecia) in a woman.

Scarring Alopecias

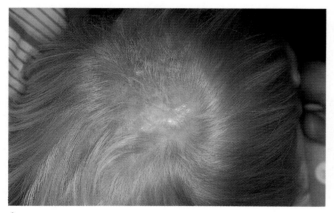

A

23.17
A, B, Aplasia cutis congenita.

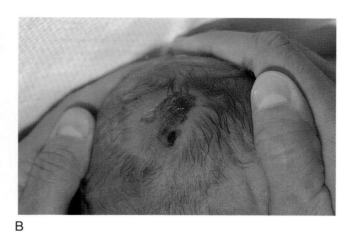

B

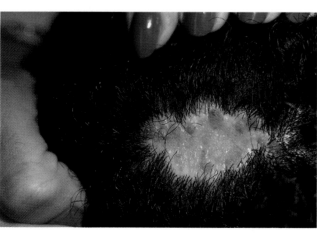

23.18
Nevus sebaceus of Jadassohn.

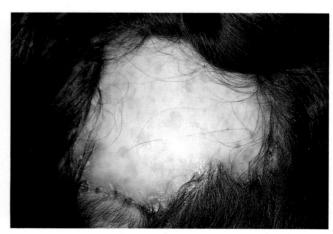

23.19
Folliculitis decalvans.

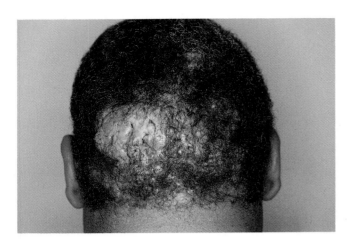

23.20
Dissecting cellulitis of the scalp.

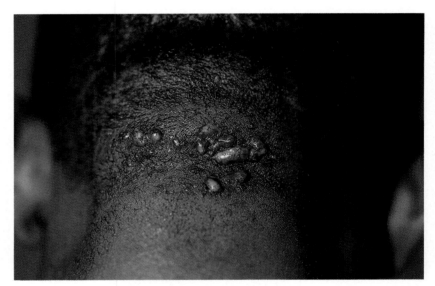

23.21
Acne keloidalis nuchae.

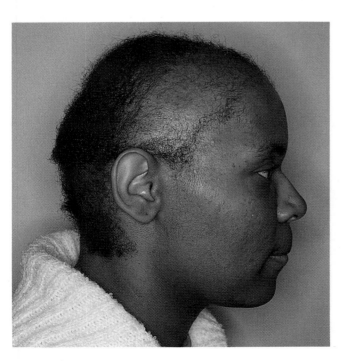

23.22
Hot comb damage resulting in scarring alopecia.

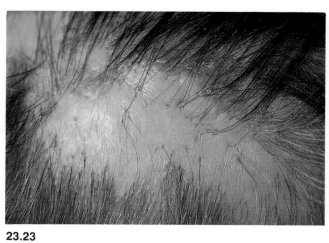

23.23
Lichen planopilaris.

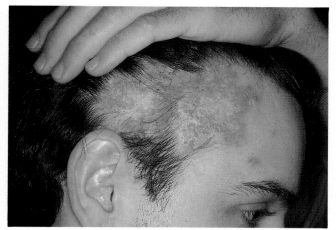

A

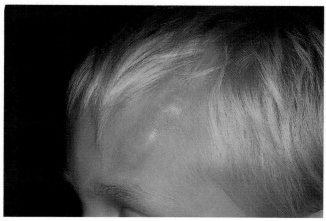

23.24
En coup de sabre. Localized linear morphea.

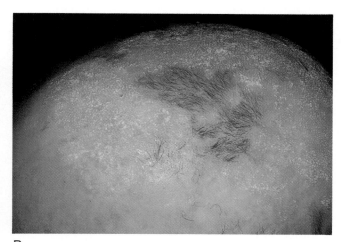

B

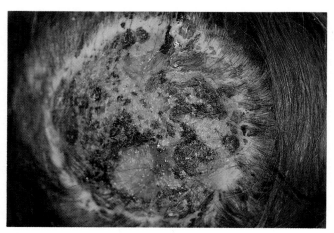

23.25
Inflammatory superficial fungal infection.

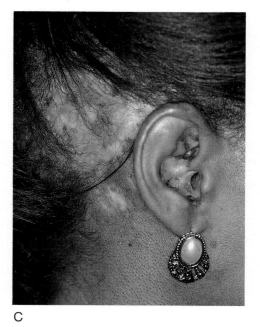

C

23.26
A to C, Discoid lupus erythematosus.

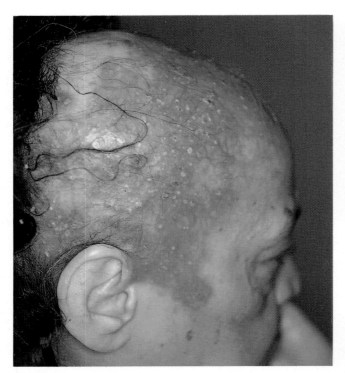

23.27
Sarcoidosis.

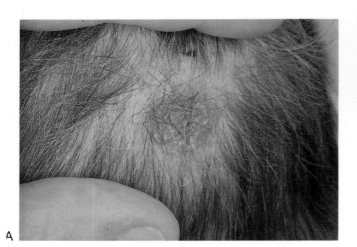

A

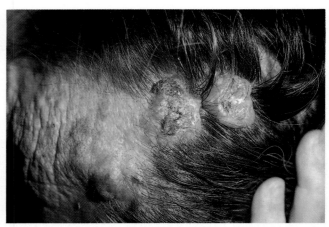

B

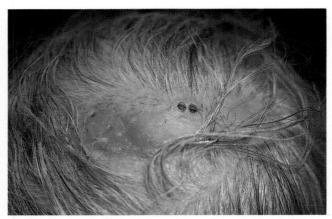

23.29
Localized cicatricial pemphigoid, Brunsting-Perry variant.

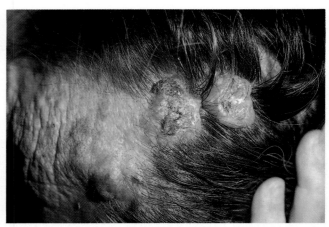

23.30
Angiosarcoma.

23.28
A, B, Metastatic lesion from squamous cell carcinoma of the lung.

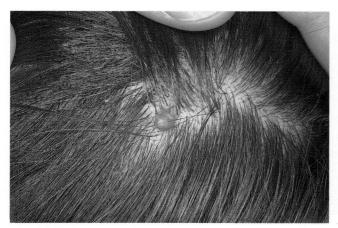

23.31
Pseudopyogenic granuloma (angiolymphoid hyperplasia with eosinophilia).

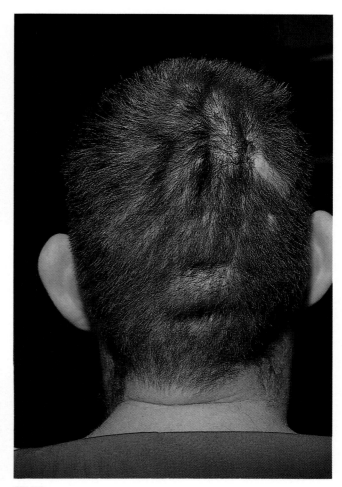

23.33
Cutis verticis gyrata.

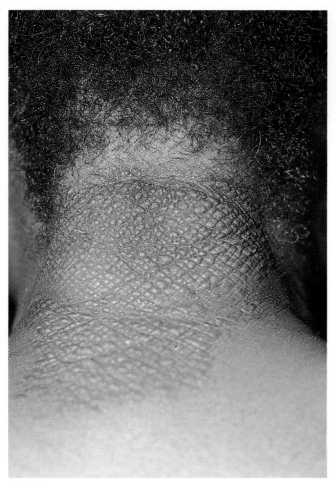

23.32
Lichen simplex chronicus.

MISCELLANEOUS HAIR DISORDERS

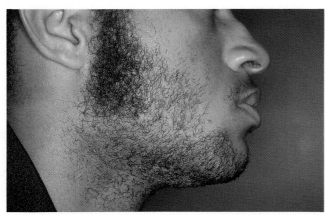

23.34
Pseudofolliculitis barbae. In this condition the natural curliness of the hair allows it to re-enter the skin next to the follicle, with a resulting inflammatory reaction.

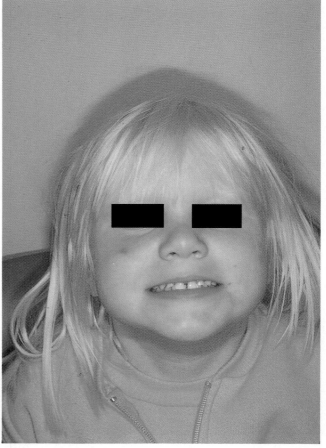

23.36
Albinism. White hair.

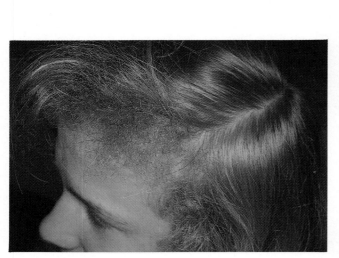

23.35
Woolly-hair nevus. A localized patch of kinky, unmanageable hair.

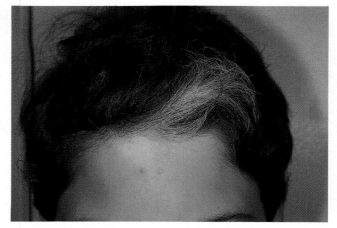

23.37
Piebaldism. White forelock.

SCALP DISORDERS

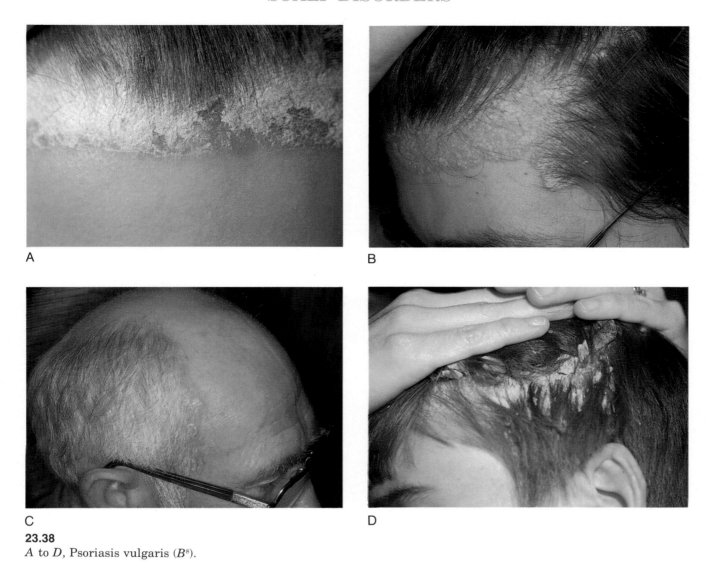

A

B

C

D

23.38
A to *D*, Psoriasis vulgaris (*B*⁸).

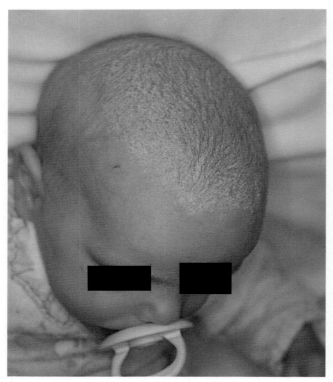

23.39
Seborrheic dermatitis in a child.

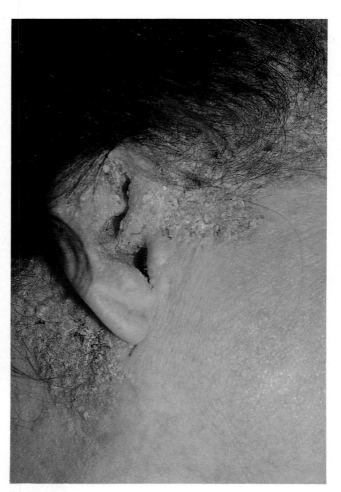

23.41
Darier's disease.

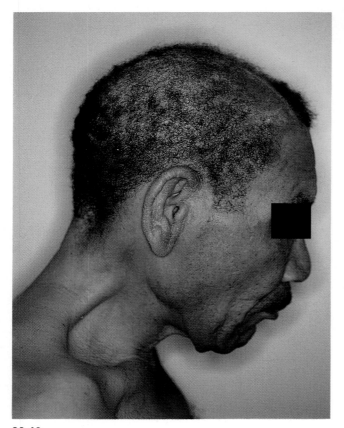

23.40
Seborrheic dermatitis in an adult.

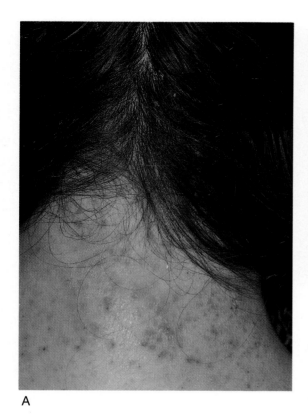

A

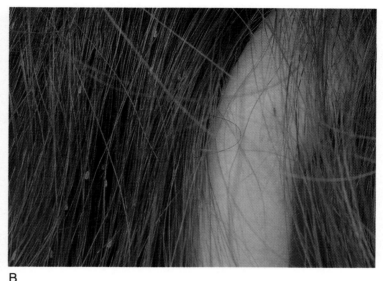

B

23.42
A, *B*, Pediculosis capitis.[2]

HYPERTRICHOSIS AND HIRSUTISM

23.43
Hypertrichosis lanuginosa.

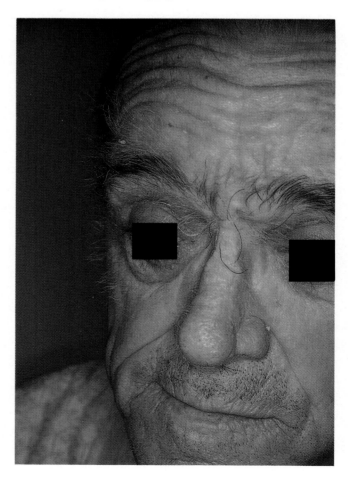

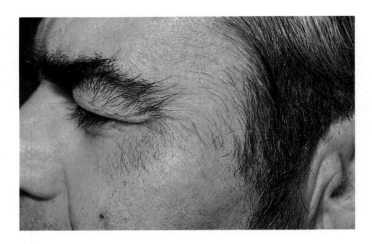

23.44
Hypertrichosis in porphyria cutanea tarda.

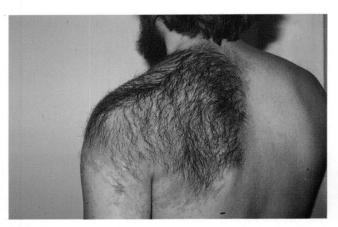

23.45
Becker's nevus.

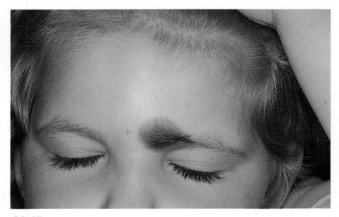

23.47
Congenital hairy nevus.

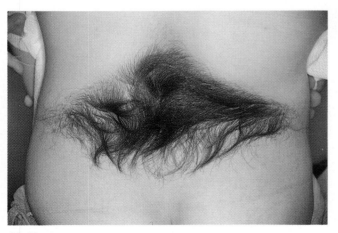

23.46
Nevus pilosus.[2]

PIGMENTARY ABNORMALITIES OF THE ORAL MUCOSA

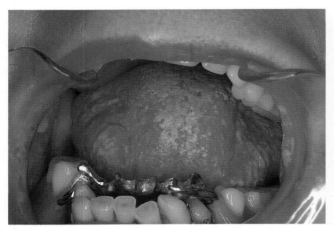

24.1
Candida albicans. White plaques on the tongue.

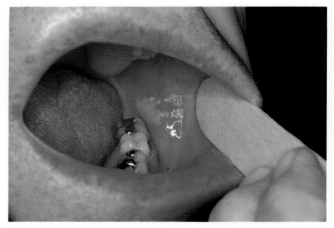

24.3
Fordyce spots on the lip (ectopic sebaceous glands).

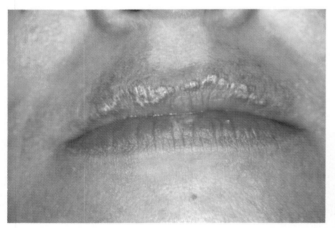

24.2
Lupus erythematosus on the lip.

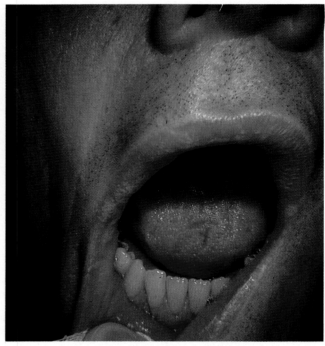

24.4
Leukoplakia. Literally this means white plaque. It may or may not represent a premalignant change.

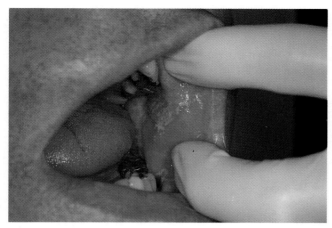

24.5
Lichen planus.

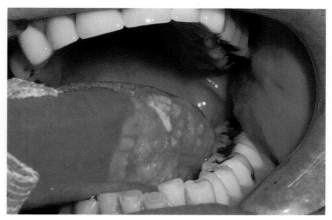

24.8
Squamous cell carcinoma.

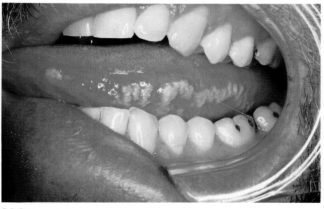

24.6
Oral hairy leukoplakia. This is a manifestation of Epstein-Barr virus infection in HIV-infected individuals.

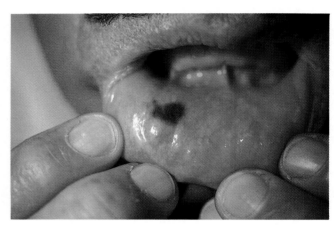

24.9
Amalgam tattoo.

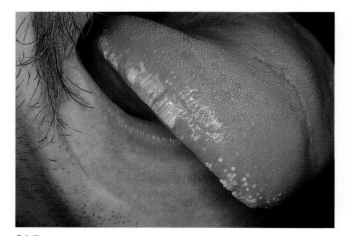

24.7
Chemical burn.

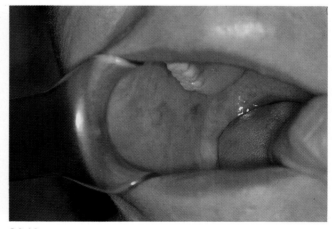

24.10
Addison's disease.

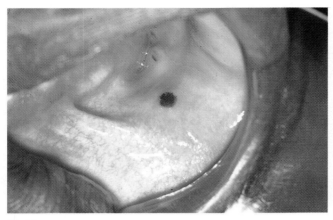

24.11
Junctional nevus of the buccal mucosa.

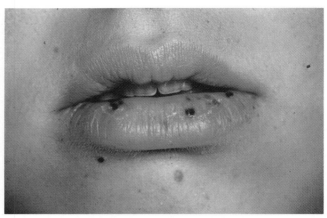

24.13
Peutz-Jeghers syndrome.[9]

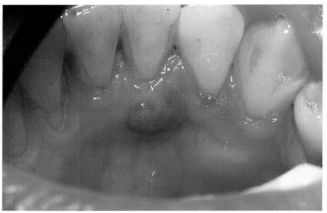

24.12
Junctional nevus.

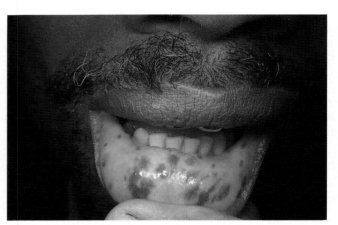

24.14
Labial melanotic macules in an HIV-infected patient.

GROWTHS

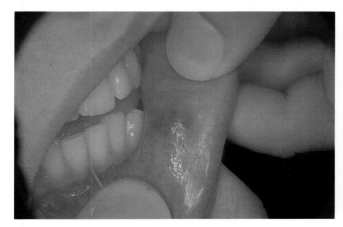

24.15
Hemangioma.

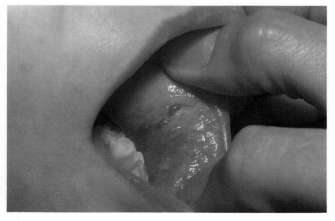

24.16
Vascular malformation (formerly cavernous hemangioma).

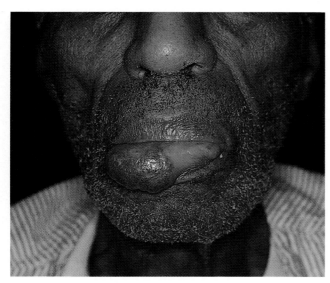

24.17
Venous lake.

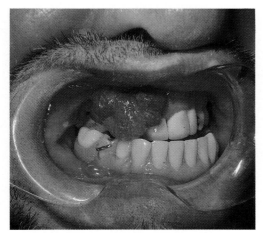

24.18
Kaposi's sarcoma.

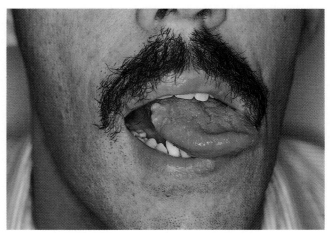

A

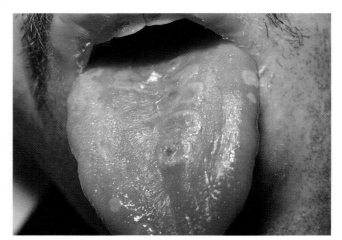

B

24.19
A, B, Verrucae vulgaris in HIV-infected men.

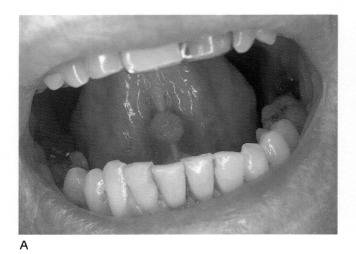

A

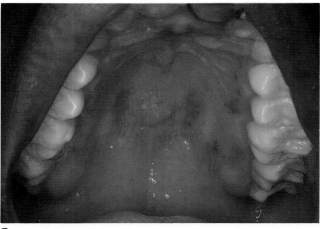

B

24.20

A, B, Condyloma acuminatum.

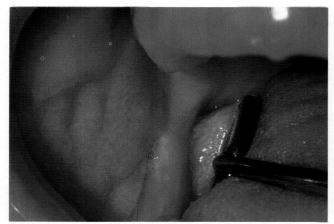

24.21

White sponge nevus.

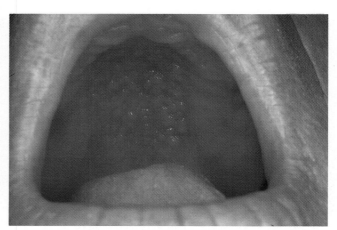

24.22

Cowden's disease (multiple hamartoma syndrome).

24.23

Palatopapillomatosis.

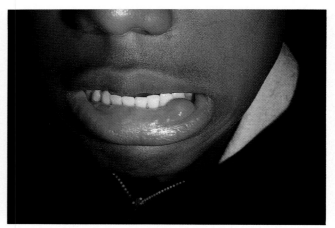

24.24

Mucocele.

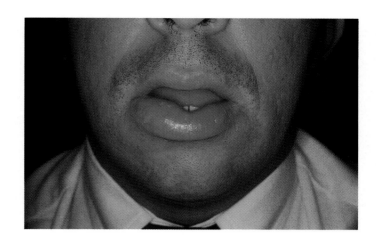

24.25
Melkersson-Rosenthal syndrome.

EROSIONS, ULCERS, BLISTERING LESIONS

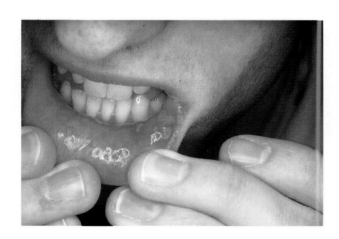

24.26
Aphthous stomatitis.

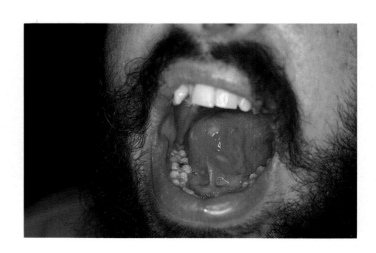

24.27
Behçet's syndrome.

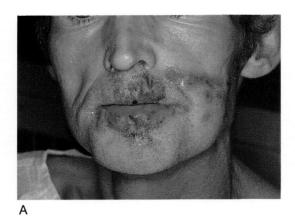

A

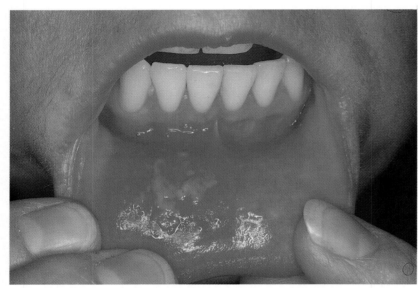

B

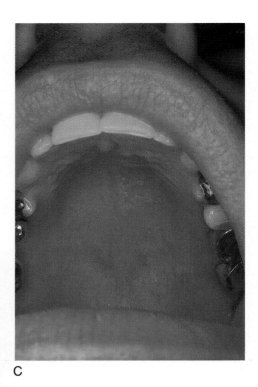

C

24.28
A to *C*, Herpes simplex.

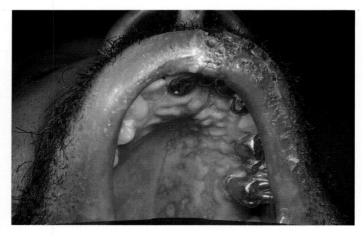

24.29
Herpes zoster in an HIV-infected individual.

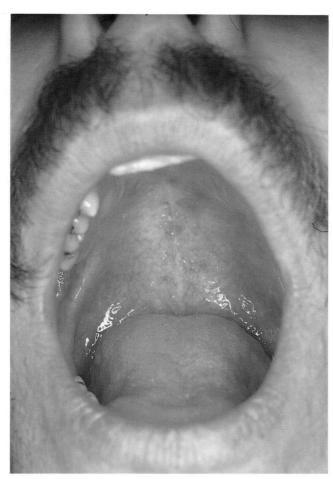

24.30
Hand-foot-and-mouth disease.

24.31
Candida albicans in an HIV-infected patient.

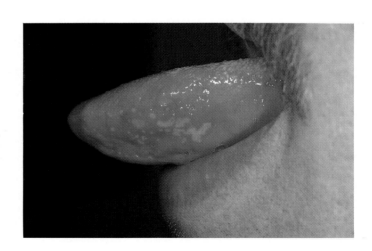

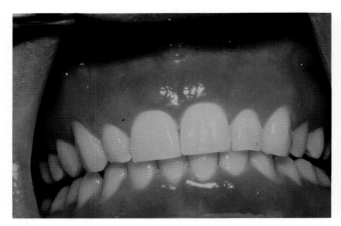

24.32
Allergic gingivitis.

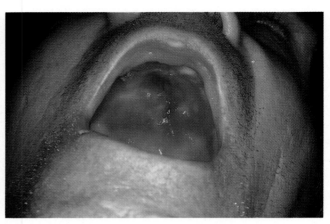

24.35
Lethal midline granuloma.

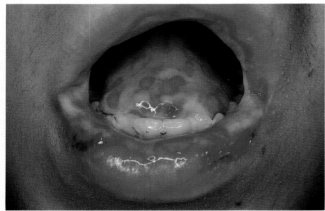

24.33
Erythema multiforme.

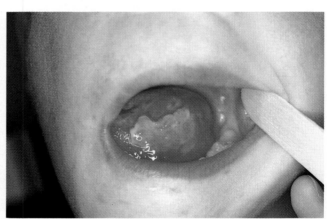

24.36
Dyskeratosis congenita.

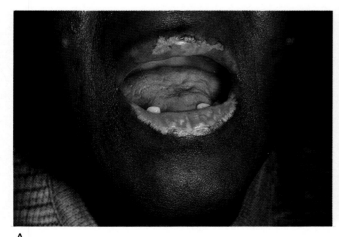

A

24.34
A, B, Discoid lupus erythematosus.

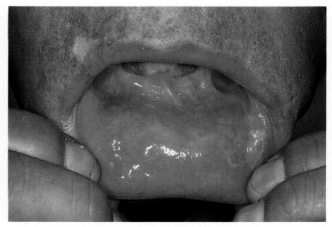

B

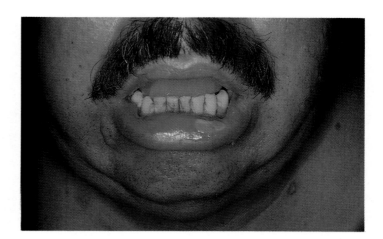

24.37
Pemphigus vulgaris.

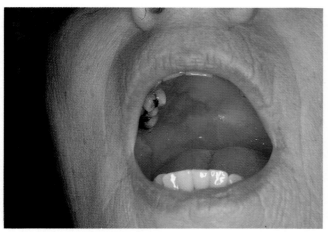

A

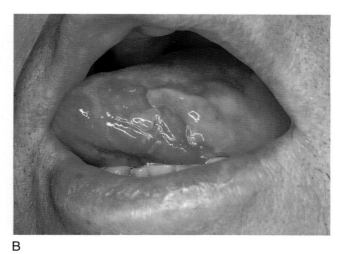

B

24.38
A, B, Cicatricial pemphigoid (benign mucous membrane pemphigoid).

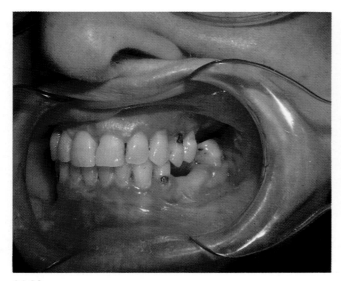

24.39
Bullous pemphigoid.

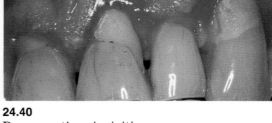

24.40
Desquamative gingivitis.

TONGUE LESIONS

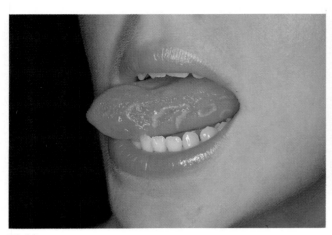

24.41
Geographic tongue.

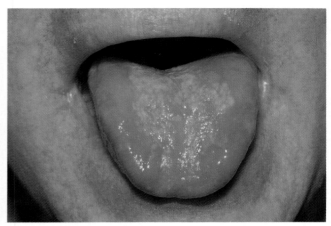

24.43
Dyskeratosis congenita.

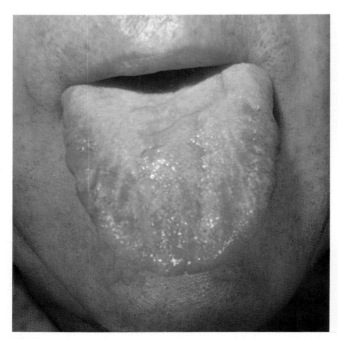

24.42
Reiter's syndrome.

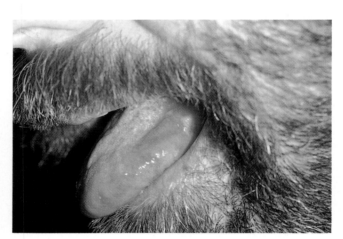

24.44
Candida albicans in an HIV-infected patient.

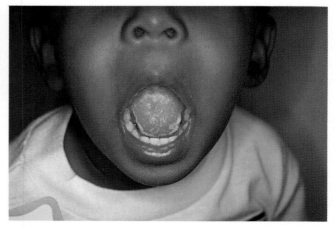

24.45
Chronic mucocutaneous candidiasis.

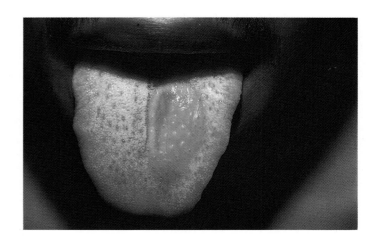

24.46
Fixed drug eruption.[12]

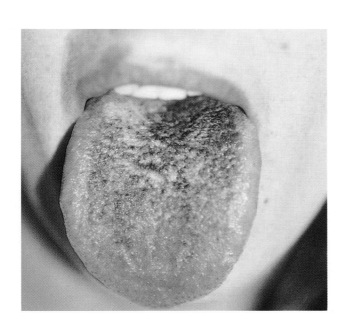

24.47
Black hairy tongue.

24.48
Scrotal tongue (lingua plicata).

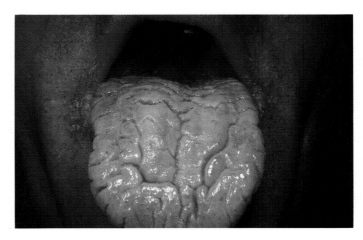

REFERENCES

Callen JP, Jorizzo J, Greer KE, Penneys N, Piette W, Zone JJ: Dermatological Signs of Internal Disease. WB Saunders Co, Philadelphia, 1988.

Champion RH, Burton JL, Ebling FJG (eds): Textbook of Dermatology. 5th ed. Blackwell Scientific Publications, London, 1992.

Fitzpatrick TB, Eisen AZ, Wolff K, Freedberg IM, Austen KF (eds): Dermatology in General Medicine. 4th ed. McGraw-Hill Book Co, New York, 1991.

Harber LC, Bickers DR: Photosensitivity Diseases. 2nd ed. BC Decker, Toronto, 1989.

der Kaloustian VM, Kurban AK: Genetic Diseases of the Skin. Springer-Verlag, Berlin, 1979.

Lazarus GS, Goldsmith LA: Diagnosis of Skin Disease. FA Davis Co, Philadelphia, 1980.

Lookingbill DP, Marks JG Jr: Principles of Dermatology. WB Saunders Co, Philadelphia, 1986.

Sams WM Jr, Lynch PJ: Principles and Practice of Dermatology. Churchill Livingstone, New York, 1990.

APPENDIX I

GENODERMATOSES

Autosomal dominant
Albright's syndrome 2.10
Basal cell nevus syndrome 3.26, 21.33
Cowden's disease (multiple hamartoma syndrome) 3.28, 24.22
Darier's disease (keratosis follicularis) 3.154, 19.14, 22.27, 23.41, Table III
Epidermolysis bullosa
    Dominant dystrophic 7.6, 21.18, Table V
    Dowling-Meara 5.29, 7-8
    Weber-Cockayne 5.29, Table V
Erythrokeratodermia variabilis 15.6, Table XI
Gardner's syndrome 4.1
Hailey-Hailey disease (chronic benign familial pemphigus) 7.17, 20.11, Table III
Hereditary generalized lentigines 2.20
Hereditary hemorrhagic telangiectasia (Osler-Weber-Rendu syndrome) 8.16, 21.24
Hypohidrotic ectodermal dysplasia 23.1, 23.2
Hypomelanosis of Ito (incontinentia pigmenti achromians) 2.47, 14.17, 18.20
Ichthyosis vulgaris 18.27, Table XI
LEOPARD syndrome 2.22
Monilethrix 23.3, 23.4
Nail-patella syndrome 22.1
Neurofibromatosis
    Café au lait spots 2.9
    Multiple neurofibromas 3.1
Pachyonychia congenita 22.24
Peutz-Jeghers syndrome 2.21, 24.13

Pili torti 23.5
Tuberous sclerosis 2.50, 3.25, 3.34, 3.74, 4.27, 22.37, 22.38
Unna-Thost palmoplantar keratoderma 21.28
Vohwinkel's palmoplantar keratoderma (mutilating keratoderma) 21.29

Autosomal recessive
Acrodermatitis enteropathica 6.5, 7.25, 8.34, 20.30
Albinism 2.46, 23.36
Ataxia telangiectasia Table VII
Bloom's syndrome 8.37, Table VII
Congenital ichthyosiform erythroderma
    Nonbullous Table XI
    Bullous Table XI
    Sjögren-Larsson syndrome Table XI
    Netherton's syndrome Table XI, 23.7
    IBIDS syndrome Table XI
Epidermodysplasia verruciformis 16.5
Epidermolysis bullosa Table V
    Dystrophic inversa 7.11, Table V
    Junctional type (generalized atrophic benign 7.7, Table V
    Junctional type (Herlitz or gravis) 7.5, Table V
    Recessive dystrophic Table V
Lamellar ichthyosis 18.29, 21.31, Table XI
Papillon-Lefèvre syndrome 21.30
Werner's syndrome 8.29
Xeroderma pigmentosum 2.6, Table VII

389

X-linked

Hypohidrotic ectodermal dysplasia 23.1, 23.2
Dyskeratosis congenita 2.14, 17.5, 22.2, 24.36, 24.43
Fabry's disease 3.103, 20.35, 21.27
Incontinentia pigmenti 2.16, 2.47, 3.148, 14.16, 14.17, 18.19, 18.20, Table III
X-linked ichthyosis 18.28, Table XI

Variable pattern

Chondrodysplasia punctata Table XI
Ehlers-Danlos syndrome Type IV 9.2
Pseudoxanthoma elasticum 3.117, 20.24

CUTANEOUS INFECTIONS

Bacterial
Actinomycosis 6.10, 10.28
Atypical mycobacterial infection 4.35, 10.19, 14.22
Bacillary angiomatosis 3.83
Cat-scratch disease 6.12
Chancroid 10.38
Erythrasma 2.11, 20.4
Gonorrhea 6.4, 9.18
Granuloma inguinale 10.39
Leprosy 2.61, 10.3
Lymphogranuloma venereum 20.47
Meningococcemia 9.19
Pseudomonas 3.51, 6.15, 22.20
Rocky Mountain spotted fever 9.23, 21.13
Staphylococcal infections 1.9, 4.34, 5.21, 5.22, 6.11, 8.13, 22.31
Tuberculosis 10.42

Viral
Exanthem 2.80, 3.54, 18.14
Fifth disease (erythema infectiosum) 2.84, 17.12
Hand-foot-and-mouth disease 5.36, 21.15, 24.30
Herpes simplex 5.32, 10.40, 10.41, 16.6, 16.8, 20.48, 21.26, 24.28
Herpes zoster 5.35, 14.11, 16.7, 18.23, 24.29
Infectious mononucleosis 2.81
Milker's nodule 4.36, 21.23
Molluscum contagiosum 1.29, 3.8, 16.9, 20.38
Oral hairy leukoplakia 24.6

Orf 5.38, 21.22
Varicella (same virus as herpes zoster) 5.34, 5.35, 9.20, 18.22
Warts 3.15, 3.16, 3.139, 3.142, 14.3, 16.5, 20.42, 24.19, 24.20

Fungal
Blastomycosis 3.143, 6.7, 10.20
Candida 6.8, 7.1, 7.18, 20.2, 20.31, 22.5, 22.13, 22.32, 24.1, 24.31, 24.44, 24.45
Cryptococcosis 10.22
Dermatophyte infection 2.12, 3.127-30, 5.8, 6.9, 7.2, 7.3, 13.8, 20.3, 22.6, 22.22, 23.15, 23.25
Sporotrichosis 10.21, 14.21
Tinea nigra palmaris 2.41
Tinea versicolor 2.31, 2.65, 3.164

Infestations
Cutaneous larva migrans 1.18, 15.1
Leishmaniasis 10.24, 14.23
Pediculosis 20.50, 23.42
Scabies 3.52, 3.167, 4.56, 5.9, 7.35, 11.16, 18.12, 20.39, 21.11, 21.12

Spirochetes
Lyme disease 8.8, 13.4
Syphilis 2.33, 3.49, 3.163, 10.37, 12.23, 13.5, 20.41, 21.10

APPENDIX III

CUTANEOUS CHANGES ASSOCIATED WITH HIV INFECTION

Bacillary angiomatosis 3.83
Candida albicans 24.31, 24.44
Cryptococcosis 10.22
Fungal granuloma 16.14
Herpes simplex 10.40, 20.48
Herpes zoster 24.29

Kaposi's sarcoma 2.73, 24.18
Labial melanotic macules 24.14
Oral hairy leukoplakia 24.6
Reiter's syndrome 22.26
Seborrheic dermatitis 23.40
Warts 24.19

APPENDIX IV

CUTANEOUS MALIGNANCIES

INDEX

Note: Pages in *italics* indicate illustrations; those followed by t refer to tables.